The Biology of
Entamoeba histolytica

TROPICAL MEDICINE RESEARCH STUDIES SERIES
Series Editor: **Dr. K. N. Brown**
National Institute for Medical Research, England

1. Schistosoma Mansoni: The Parasite Surface in Relation to Host Immunity
   Diane J. McLaren

2. The Biology of *Entamoeba histolytica*
   Adolfo Martínez-Palomo

The Biology of *Entamoeba histolytica*

Adolfo Martínez-Palomo, M.D.,D.Sc.

*Head, Department of Cell Biology and
Section of Experimental Parasitology,
Centro de Investigación y de Estudios
Avanzados del Instituto Politécnico Nacional,
Mexico City, Mexico*

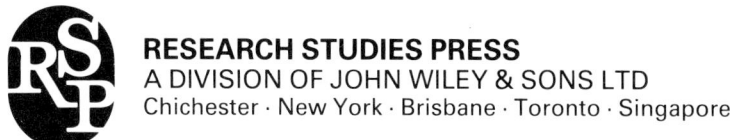

RESEARCH STUDIES PRESS
A DIVISION OF JOHN WILEY & SONS LTD
Chichester · New York · Brisbane · Toronto · Singapore

RESEARCH STUDIES PRESS

Editorial Office:
58B Station Road, Letchworth, Herts. SG6 3BE, England

Copyright ©1982, by John Wiley & Sons Ltd.

All rights reserved.

No part of this book may be reproduced by any means, nor transmitted, nor translated into a machine language without the written permission of the publisher.

British Library Cataloguing in Publication Data:

Martínez-Palomo, Adolfo
   The Biology of *entamoeba histolytica*.—(Tropical medicine research studies series)
   1. Amebiasis
   I. Title   II. Series
   593.1'17   QR201.A/
   ISBN 0 471 10404 3

Printed in Great Britain

To Rosamaría

Table of Contents

Table of Contents	vii
Preface	xi
1. INTRODUCTION	1
2. CELL BIOLOGY	
2.1 The Trophozoite: Cell Form and Motility	5
2.2 The Cytoplasm	11
2.2.1 Vacuolar system	11
2.2.2 Tubular system	17
2.2.3 Ribosomal helical arrays	19
2.2.4 Cytoskeleton	25
2.2.5 Cylindrical bodies	27
2.2.6 Filamentous and polyhedral viruses	31
2.3 The Cell Surface	32
2.3.1 The surface coat	32
2.3.2 The plasma membrane	35
2.3.3 Capping	38
2.3.4 Shedding	40
2.3.5 Dense oval bodies	41
2.3.6 Surface specializations	42
2.4 The Nucleus	50
2.5 The Cyst	56

3. BIOCHEMISTRY	61
3.1 Anaerobic and Aerobic Metabolism	61
3.2 Membrane Composition	65
3.3 Growth and Differentiation	68
4. SPECIES OF *ENTAMOEBA*	73
4.1 Strain Variations	76
4.1.1 The unicist hypothesis	76
4.1.2 The dualistic hypothesis	77
4.1.3 The pluralistic hypothesis	78
4.2 *Entamoeba histolytica*-like Amebas	79
4.3 Differences Between Carrier and Invasive Strains	80
4.4 Biochemical Taxonomy	81
5. IMMUNOLOGY OF AMEBIASIS[*]	85
5.1 Characterization of Amebic Antigens	85
5.2 Subcellular Location of Amebic Antigens	87
5.3 Humoral Immune Reactions	88
5.4 Possible Means of Evasion of the Humoral Immune Response	90
5.5 Cellular Immune Reactions	91
5.6 Resistance to Reinfection	93
5.7 Induction of Protective Immunity	93
6. PARASITE FACTORS OF VIRULENCE	95
6.1 Virulence of Pathogenic Strains	96
6.2 Viruses and Virulence	98
6.3 Virulence and Culture Conditions	99
6.3.1 Bacterial associates	99
6.3.2 Cholesterol	101
6.3.3 Number of passages in culture	101
6.3.4 Strain heterogeneity	102
6.4 Attachment	103
6.5 Multiplication and Penetration	105
6.6 Evasion of Host Defenses	108
6.7 Cytotoxicity	109
6.7.1 Toxins in homogenates of trophozoites	109
6.7.2 Contact-dependent cytopathic effect	110

[*]In collaboration with Dr. B. Sepúlveda

7.	SOME UNSOLVED PROBLEMS IN AMEBIASIS RELATED TO THE BIOLOGY OF THE PARASITE	119
8.	REFERENCES	123
9.	SELECTED MONOGRAPHS AND ARTICLES ON AMEBIASIS	155
	9.1 History of Amebiasis	155
	9.2 Clinical Aspects of Amebiasis	157
10.	INDEX	159

Preface

The creation of the Centro de Estudios sobre Amibiasis (Center for the Study of Amebiasis) in Mexico during the last decade gave rise to a renewed interest in an important, often neglected, and frequently misunderstood human disease. As a result of the tireless activity of its founder, Dr. Bernardo Sepúlveda, the Center has offered continuous support for the realization of interdisciplinary medical research on subjects ranging from the molecular biology of *Entamoeba histolytica* to the improvement of diagnostic and therapeutic procedures and the study of the epidemiology and prophylaxis of amebiasis. The constant support and advice received from the members of the Center, and particularly from Dr. Sepúlveda, are gratefully acknowledged. I have also greatly benefited from the numerous and stimulating discussions with Dr. Manuel Martínez-Báez and Dr. Louis S. Diamond, and with my colleagues Dr. Miguel Tanimoto, Dr. Rubén López-Revilla, Dr. Jesús Calderón, Dr. Jorge Cerbón, and Dr. Víctor Tsutsumi.

The writing of this monograph and the original research described herein were made possible through the support of Dr. Manuel V. Ortega, Director of the Center for Research and Advanced Studies of the National Polytechnic Institute of Mexico, Dr. Federico Chávez Peón, Undersecretary of Health of Mexico, Dr. Kenneth S. Warren, Director of the Health Sciences Division of the Rockefeller Foundation, U.S.A., and Dr. Gonzalo Gutiérrez-Trujillo, Head of the Division of Education and Research of the Mexican Institute for Social Security. I am also grateful to Dr. Gaetan Tremblay, Head of the Department of Pathology of the University of Montreal, Canada, for his hospitality during the summer of 1980.

The monograph was written during three summer periods, two of them spent at Bethesda, Maryland, U.S.A., and one at Montreal, Canada. The first two periods were funded with a grant from the Guggenheim Foundation, and the third with a grant from the Rockefeller Foundation. The services of the National Library of Medicine, U.S.A., and the Library of Medicine of the University of Montreal, Canada, were fundamental for the completion of this work. Dr. K.N. Brown has made possible the publication of this book and has kindly reviewed the text. The original research described was partially supported by grants from the National Council for Science and Technology (CONACyT), Mexico, and the Rockefeller Foundation (Great Neglected Diseases of Mankind Network).

Studies on the ultrastructure of *E. histolytica* were carried out with the invaluable collaboration of Arturo González-Robles and Bibiana Chávez. Work on experimental amebiasis was done with Dr. Miguel Tanimoto, and Margarita de la Torre was responsible for the isolation, axenization, and cultivation of most of the strains of *E. histolytica* used in our experiments. I have received continuous stimulus from past or present students interested in experimental amebiasis, among them, Dr. Arnulfo Cervantes, Dr. Esther Orozco, Carlos Argüello, Fernando Anaya, and Raúl Mena. The patient and skillful typing and retyping of the manuscript by Mrs. Verónica Dueñas was particularly helpful. I am particularly indebted to Dr. M. Martínez-Báez, Dr. Bernardo Sepúlveda, Dr. K.N. Brown, Dr. L.S. Diamond, and Dr. C. Mackenzie for reviewing parts of the manuscript.

The editorial assistance of Ms. Marcella Vogt is gratefully acknowledged.

CHAPTER 1
Introduction

Amebiasis is the infection of man with the intestinal protozoan parasite *Entamoeba histolytica* Schaudinn, 1903. This species usually lives as a commensal in the lumen of the large intestine (lumenal amebiasis), but may invade the intestinal mucosa producing dysentery or ameboma; through blood-borne spreading, it can give rise to extraintestinal lesions, particularly in the liver (invasive amebiasis).

The parasite was found by Lesh in 1875 in a patient from Archangel, near the Arctic Circle, who suffered chronic dysentery associated with the presence of amebas in his stools. Although these amebas produced dysentery when inoculated into a dog, Lesh did not believe that the parasite was the causative agent. The pathogenic role of the amebas was demonstrated by various investigators, notably by Kartulis (1887) working in Egypt, who additionally described the existence of amebic liver lesions. In 1891, Councilman and Lafleur provided detailed pathological and clinical descriptions of amebic dysentery and amebic liver abscesses. Walker and Sellards (1913) conclusively demonstrated in the Philippines that *Entamoeba coli* was nonpathogenic and *E. histolytica* was pathogenic. As the details of the life cycle of the parasite were unraveled, other species and genera of amebas were found living as commensals in the human gastrointestinal tract, and *E. histolytica* was frequently reported in humans lacking dysenteric symptoms and lesions. Rough estimates indicated that in certain warm climatic regions, the trophozoites of *E. histolytica* gave rise to invasive amebiasis in one out of every five infected persons, whereas in temperate regions, infection was accompanied by clinical signs in only one of every two million cases. This situation prompted Brumpt (1925, 1949) to establish a new species of ameba ("*E. dispar*") characterized by its innocuousness, in contrast to the morphologically indistinguishable but pathogenic "*E. dysenteriae*", a proposal that was not accepted by protozoologists.

As a consequence of these uncertainties, great confusion has prevailed for decades with regard to the significance of the parasitological diagnosis of intestinal infection with *E. histolytica*. The presence of *E. histolytica* in feces, whose identification requires considerable experience and thus may frequently be mistaken, has been taken as an indication for vigorous chemotherapy, probably without justification in many cases, with the consequent production of iatrogenic damage in some patients, since amebicidal drugs, although generally effective, are potentially toxic. Efforts to clarify this situation led protozoologists to the classification of *E. hartmanni*, formerly known as the "small race" of *E. histolytica*, as a distinct species, and to the more recent recognition of the existence of pathogenic and nonpathogenic strains of *E. histolytica*, the former displaying a wide range of virulence.

Invasive amebiasis is still a major health and social problem in various regions of the world where inadequate sanitary conditions together with poverty, ignorance, and crowding, and the prevalence of highly virulent strains combine to sustain a high incidence of intestinal amebiasis in children of all ages, and of liver abscesses in adults, usually males. Both forms may be fatal unless prompt diagnosis is followed by adequate treatment. In temperate zones where affluent societies prevail, the number of severe cases of invasive amebiasis is much lower. Nevertheless, knowledge of the disease in these regions is also important because: a) failure to identify the nature of an amebic infection may have a fatal outcome; b) high infection rates occur among certain immigrant groups; c) epidemic outbreaks in institutions such as schools or mental hospitals are possible; and d) there is a recently discovered, apparently elevated incidence of lumenal amebiasis among male homosexuals.

During the last decade, there has been an upsurge in the number of investigations on amebiasis as a result of various factors, among them: the recognition of the need to study the basic aspects of the biology of this potentially lethal, relatively common parasite; the establishment of multidisciplinary centers for the study of amebiasis by Elsdon-Dew in South Africa, and by Sepúlveda in

Mexico; and the introduction of the first practical method for the axenic cultivation of *E. histolytica* by Diamond in 1968. This current interest in amebiasis has occurred in spite of the unexplained failure of international health organizations to recognize, until very recently, the need for better knowledge of the disease.

As a result of recent investigations concerning some basic aspects of the biology of the parasite, information on the fine structure, biochemistry, in vitro cultivation, and strain differences of *E. histolytica* has considerably increased. The analysis of virulence factors has given new insight into the mechanisms by which the ameba invades and destroys mammalian tissues while avoiding the immune response of the host. Investigations on the immunology of human and experimental amebiasis have led to new methods for the serological diagnosis of invasive amebiasis and have suggested the possible existence of protective immunity following invasive infections. The present monograph represents an attempt to critically review these issues and to summarize the significant results from the vast, complex, and conflicting literature that spans more than a century. While the search for references was intended to be comprehensive, regardless of language or date of publication, the references given in the text represent only that small fraction which the author considers to contain valuable information. Other monographs on subjects such as history, epidemiology, pathology, immunology, and clinical aspects of the disease, are listed separately. The relatively large number of original illustrations reflects not only the author's background and interests, but also are a consequence of the fact that the ultrastructural study of the parasite and its interaction with host tissues has been the most prolific topic of biomedical research in amebiasis for the last twenty years.

This monograph was written because it was felt that at present, as various research groups are introducing the modern weapons of cellular and molecular biology and immunology to the study of amebiasis, a review was needed in order to evaluate the present status of our knowledge of the biology of the parasite, dispersed in books, journals, and proceedings of unrelated medical and biological specialties.

CHAPTER 2
Cell Biology

2.1 The Trophozoite: Cell Form and Motility

The trophozoite or motile form of *E. histolytica* is a highly dynamic and pleomorphic cell whose form and motility are extremely sensitive to changes in the physicochemical environment. Cooling below 37° C results in progressive sluggishness; amebas become spherical and detach from the substrate, while those that form clumps tend to disaggregate. Local variations in pH, osmolarity, and redox potential may also alter the form and motility of the cells. A pleomorphic shape, active motility, and attachment to the culture flask or to other amebas to form clusters are excellent indicators of the viability of cultured trophozoites. Under adverse conditions such as are found in old cultures, spherical amebas detach from the surface of growth or cease to agglutinate with their neighbors, and show little evidence of translational and internal mobility.

Rounded trophozoites of *E. histolytica* measure between 7 and 40 μm (Figures 1 and 2). The diameter of the amebas is of practical importance as it is the main criterion by which *E. histolytica* can be differentiated from the smaller, nonpathogenic *Entamoeba hartmanni*. However, this situation is complicated by the fact that variations in size are not only related to strain differences, but also to feeding conditions. Amebas obtained directly from liver or intestinal lesions are generally large, measuring about 20–40 μm in diameter, while those found in nondysenteric stools or in cultures measure 7–30 μm. Furthermore, the diameter of living trophozoites tends to be larger than that of fixed amebas stained with Heidenhain's hematoxylin, due to shrinkage induced by fixation.

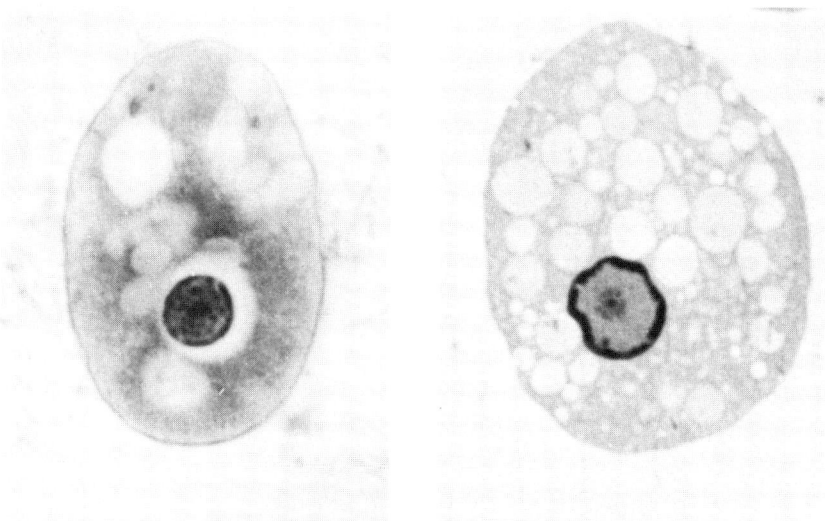

Figure 1. Trophozoite of *E. histolytica* obtained from dysenteric stools. Heidenhein's hematoxylin staining. X 1,200.

Figure 2. Trophozoite obtained from an axenic culture. Toluidine blue staining. X 1,200.

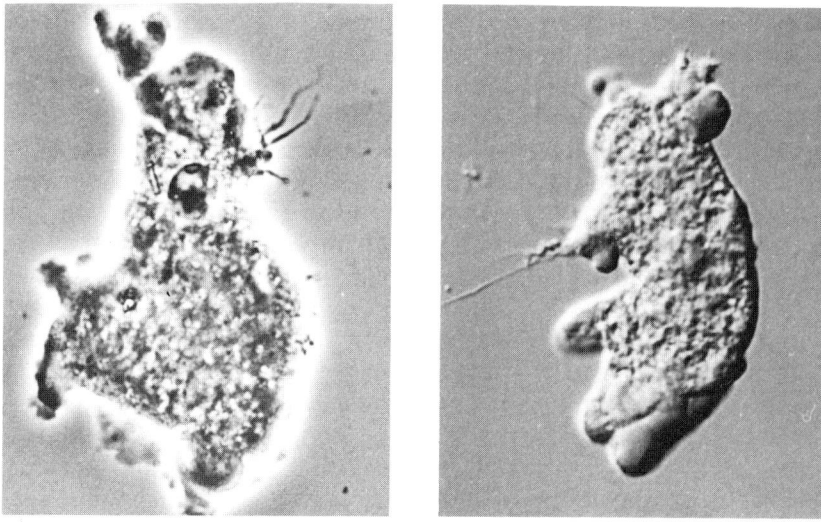

Figure 3. Phase contrast micrograph of a trophozoite. X 1,200.

Figure 4. Light micrograph of a trophozoite using Nomarski optics. X 1,200.

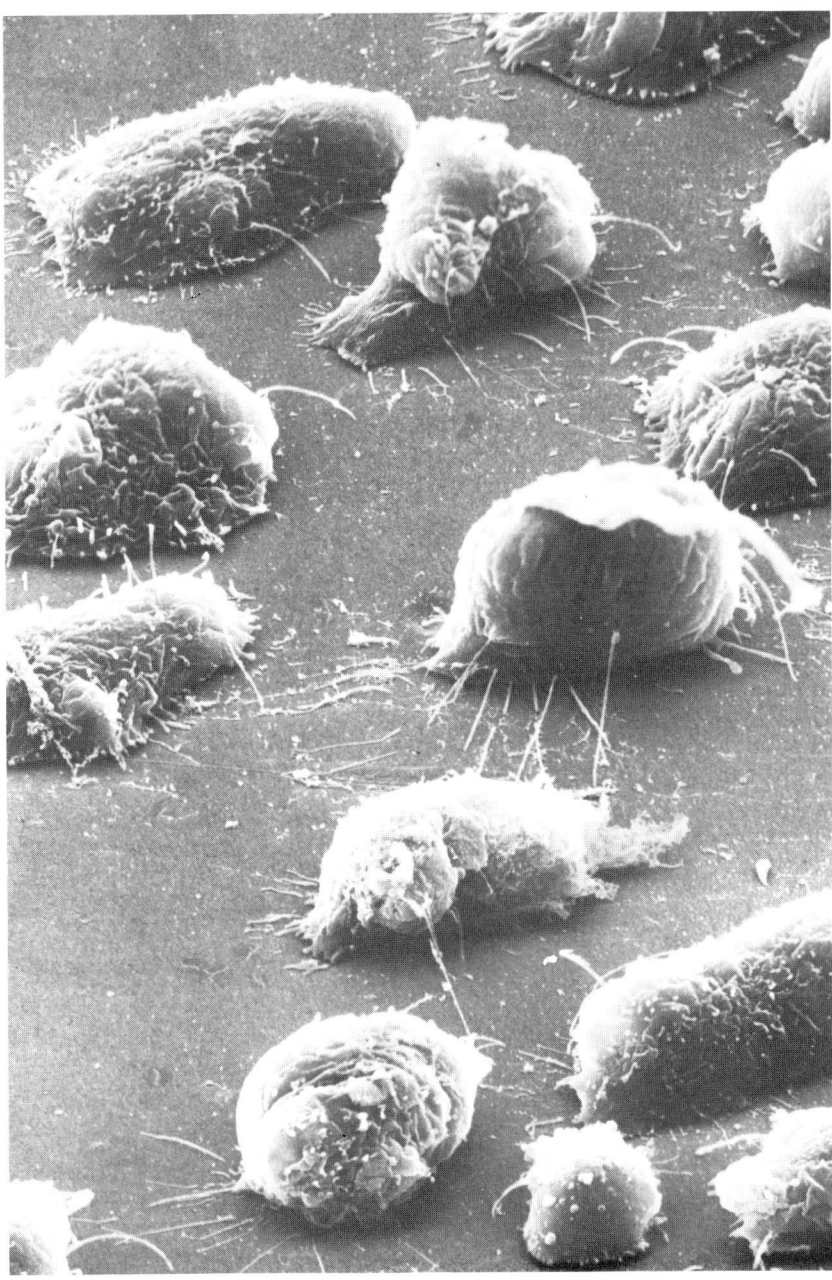

Figure 5. Scanning electron micrograph of cultured trophozoites, HK9 strain. Abundant filopodia are present. X 1,000.

In histological sections of tissues containing trophozoites, amebas appear to be spherical and are surrounded by a clear halo, interpreted as evidence of the lytic activity of the parasite. However, amebas do not have a halo in adequately fixed specimens; this phenomenon is due to cellular shrinkage from poor fixation such as occurs using formalin. Living trophozoites can be studied under the light microscope with phase contrast (Figure 3) or Nomarski differential interference optics (Figure 4).

The extreme pleomorphism of the trophozoites of *E. histolytica* is evident when they are examined with the scanning electron microscope, which best reveals their shape and surface morphology (Figures 5-7). When preservation is adequate, practically every cell has a shape different from that of its neighbors. In general, amebas are elongate in form, with protruding lobopodia and a trailing uroid. Less active cells tend to be spherical, without lobopodia or a uroid, and with varying amounts of small and large surface openings. Most of the cell surface has a wrinkled appearance, with circular openings ranging from 0.2 to 0.4 μm in diameter that correspond to the mouths of micropinocytic vesicles (Figure 6). Protruding stomas of macropinocytic channels are much larger, ranging from 2 to 6 μm in diameter (Figure 7). These structures have a smooth surface and micropinocytotic vesicles are absent. One or several finger-like lobopodia may also be found with a smooth surface. When present, the uroid appears as a tail formed by irregular folds of the membrane and filiform processes or filopodia. Amebas in contact with epithelial tissues have abundant filopodia. According to Lushbaugh and Pittman (1979), filopodia may be found at any site on the cell surface, although the majority are associated with the uroid.

Rapid directional locomotion is characteristic of trophozoites of *E. histolytica* obtained from freshly passed stools examined at temperatures approaching 37°C. Under these conditions, amebas move in one direction in a slug-like manner, without a clear distinction between endoplasm and ectoplasm (Dobell 1919). According to Deschiens (1965), trophozoites may move at a speed of 50 μm per second. As cells cool to room temperature, their motility decreases and large hyaline ectoplasmic pseudopodia, clearly distinct from the endoplasmic region, begin to appear. These finger-like, smoothly contoured lobopodia are explosively extruded. Once the trophozoites cease to move over the microscope slide, peripheral pseudopodia displaying continuous circular motion appear, probably reflecting an early stage of cellular degeneration.

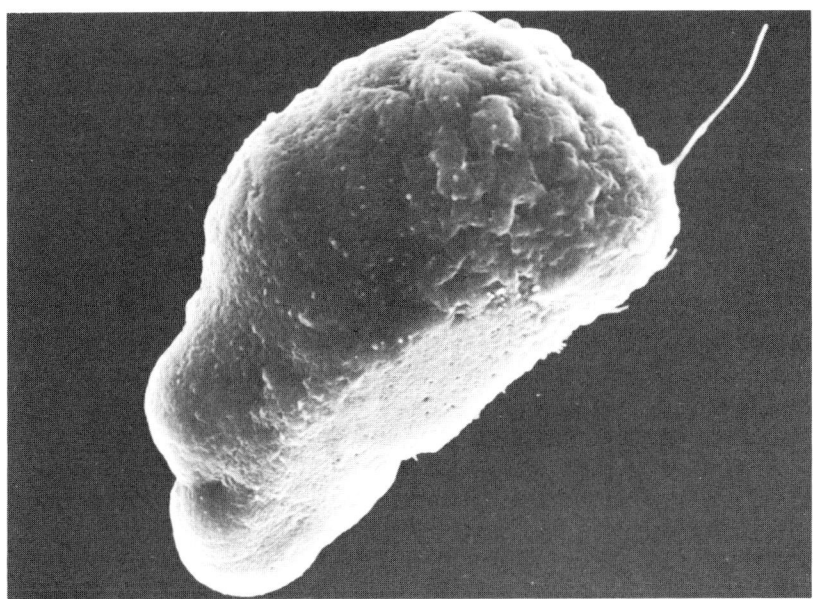

Figure 6. Scanning electron micrograph of a trophozoite showing the basal region of the detached ameba. X 2,000.

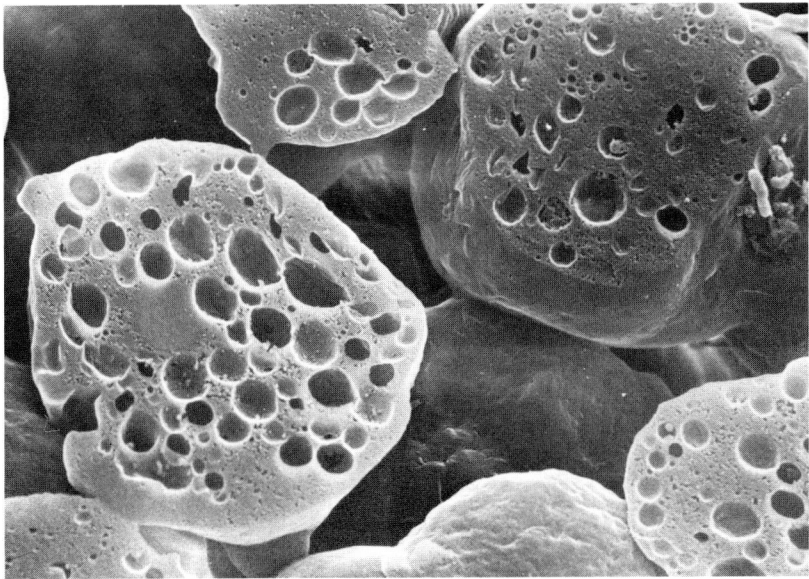

Figure 7. Scanning electron micrograph of freeze-fractured trophozoites, displaying abundant cytoplasmic vacuoles. X 1,000.

Cultured axenic trophozoites of *E. histolytica* show less pronounced locomotion. In turn, amebas in mixed cultures display more vigorous movements in comparison to axenic or monoxenic cells. Occasionally, a frontal hyaline "pseudopodium" may be found in cultured trophozoites, differing from true pseudopodia in that it is a fixed and nonmotile structure.

Actively moving trophozoites have a well-defined morphological polarity. One or several pseudopodia form and disappear rapidly at the anterior end of the protozoan, while a more permanent uroid is found at the posterior end in many active amebas. The fan-shaped uroid appears to be a region of high adhesiveness, since debris, bacteria, or cell fragments are usually attached to it. These residues are partially eliminated as the amebas slide over the substrate. Slender filopodia are generally detectable with light microscopy as trailing filamentous extensions of the uroid. When in suspension, the polarity and motility of amebas is less pronounced. In semisolid medium such as agar, trophozoites are slightly irregular in shape and show only discrete translational movements. In contrast to a total cellular displacement of a few millimeters over 2 to 3 days when in agar, amebas grown in a liquid medium on a slant may move more than 60 mm in 3 to 5 days (Snyder and Meleney 1946).

2.2 The Cytoplasm

The endoplasm of *E. histolytica* contains abundant vesicles embedded in a cytoplasmic matrix with the appearance of ground glass. Cytoplasmic vesicles in amebas from dysenteric stools may contain ingested red blood cells or food vacuoles may be filled with starch or bacteria. When present, red blood cells are the only obvious inclusions in the cytoplasm of *E. histolytica* trophozoites. The phagocytized erythrocytes may be intact or in various stages of digestion. In addition to cytoplasmic vesicles, a highly complex vacuolar and tubular system related to pinocytotic processes can be revealed by phase contrast light microscopy with the aid of time-lapse microcinematography (Chévez et al. 1971).

Trophozoites fixed at $37°C$ show an irregular profile in thin sections studied with the transmission electron microscope (Figure 8); when fixed at a lower temperature they have a circular outline. A clear-cut distinction between endoplasm and ectoplasm is found only in phagocytic or macropinocytic channels, in which the ectoplasm appears as a region of fibrogranular material of lower electron density than the endoplasm. The latter contains vacuoles and a variety of cytoplasmic particles. The difference between both regions is less striking in pseudopodia, here the ectoplasm shows an overall structure similar to the endoplasm, except for the lack of vacuoles and large particulated inclusions. The frontal hyaline "pseudopodium" occasionally found in cultures of *E. histolytica* appears as essentially devoid of cytoplasmic components under the electron microscope. It is neither a vacuole, since it is not limited by a cytoplasmic membrane, nor a pseudopodium, because it is a stable differentiation of the cell structure.

The earliest electron microscopic studies (Deutsch and Zaman 1959; Osada 1959) revealed that the submicroscopic organization of the cytoplasm of *E. histolytica* trophozoites is characterized by the absence of most of the differentiated organelles found in "typical" eukaryotic cells; i.e., mitochondria, the Golgi apparatus, rough endoplasmic reticulum, centrioles, and microtubules (Figure 8).

2.2.1 Vacuolar system

A sizeable portion of the cytoplasm of *E. histolytica* trophozoites is occupied by a heterogeneous population of membrane-limited vesicles and vacuoles, most of which have a circular profile in thin sections, with an extremely variable size ranging from 0.5 μm to more than 9.0 μm in diameter (Figures 8 and 9). In earlier ultrastructural studies, the vesicles and vacuoles in the cytoplasm of amebas were collectively termed "food vacuoles". Although there is little doubt that most of them are derived from internalized regions of the plasma membrane through various forms of endocytosis such as micro- and macropinocytosis and phagocytosis, the study of the nature and function of the vacuolar system has only recently been initiated. The membrane that limits the cytoplasmic vacuoles is approximately 10 nm thick and in thin sections resembles the plasma membrane of *E. histolytica*, except that the surface coat is facing the inside of the vacuoles, as is expected for vacuoles formed through the invagination of the cell surface. The asymmetric structure of the vacuolar membrane is also evident in freeze-fracture replicas (Figure 9) which reveal a greater quantity of membrane particles on the concave faces, in contrast to the plasma membrane, in which the convex regions have more membrane particles.

The contents of the cytoplasmic vacuoles in *E. histolytica* vary considerably according to the origin of the amebas. In trophozoites grown under axenic conditions, the vacuoles appear mostly empty under the electron microscope (Figure 8), while cellular fragments are readily identifiable in amebas grown with bacteria or other protozoa, or in amebas obtained from invasive lesions in which debris from epithelial, red blood, and inflammatory cells may be found in various stages of cellular lysis (Figure 10). The following types of vacuoles can be ultrastructurally identified in the cytoplasm of *E. histolytica*: a) phagocytic vacuoles, b) macropinocytic vacuoles, c) micropinocytic vacuoles, d) "primary lysosomes," e) "secondary lysosomes," f) residual bodies, and g) autophagic vacuoles. The first two types probably represent the same endocytic phenomenon; they are only distinguished because large particulate material is found inside phagocytic vacuoles.

There has been some controversy concerning the lysosomal nature of the cytoplasmic vacuoles of *E. histolytica* . The problem derives from the fact that in the great majority of lysosomes found in animal cells, lysosomal enzymes are unbound inside membrane-limited vacuoles. This arrangement gives rise to the characteristic structure-linked latency of lysosomal particles. In addition, the enzymes in typical lysosomes are in soluble form. In the case of the vacuoles of *E. histolytica*, cytochemical (Figure 11) and biochemical assays of isolated membrane fractions have indicated that at least one of the characteristic enzyme markers of lysosomes, acid phosphatase, is not found in soluble form, but constitutes an integral part of the membrane (Serrano et al. 1977). Eaton et al (1970), Rosenbaum and Wittner (1970), and Aley et al.(1980) observed that acid phosphatase reactivity is mainly associated with the vacuolar membrane, rather than being free in the interior of the vacuole. These findings were confirmed by Treviño-García Manzo et al.(1971) and Lushbaugh et al.(1976). If the classic definition of lysosomes is restricted to cytoplasmic particles containing a variety of hydrolases, most of which have maximal activity at acid pH and display latency in their activity if the particles are properly isolated, the term lysosome can be loosely applied to those vacuoles of *E. histolytica* that have acid phosphatase reactivity. A more rigorous interpretation of the term lysosome only serves to stimulate fruitless discussions. It remains to be determined, however, if all cytoplasmic vacuoles contain hydrolases, and to compare their enzyme content with that of well-characterized lysosomes.

The plasma membrane of the trophozoites may also contain acid phosphatase activity, as suggested by ultrastructural cytochemistry (Rondanelli et al.1977). The presence of the enzyme at the cell surface would explain the acid phosphatase reactivity found by Aley et al.(1980) in purified fractions of the plasma membrane of *E. histolytica*.

Primary lysosomes, i.e., vesicles that contain hydrolases that have not been active in molecular degradation, have not been differentiated from secondary lysosomes in amebas. Other types of lysosomes such as residual bodies and autophagic vacuoles can be easily distinguished by their ultrastructural features.

An interesting observation made by Fletcher et al.(1962) is that a given vacuole in amebas grown in mixed cultures contains only one type of food particle (bacteria, starch grains, or red blood cells), indicating the existence of several populations of phagocytic vacuoles, probably based on different binding properties of the various particles to the cell surface of the amebas. Most particles are phagocytosed singly and are transported to and collected in vacuoles where digestion takes place (Lushbaugh et al.1976).

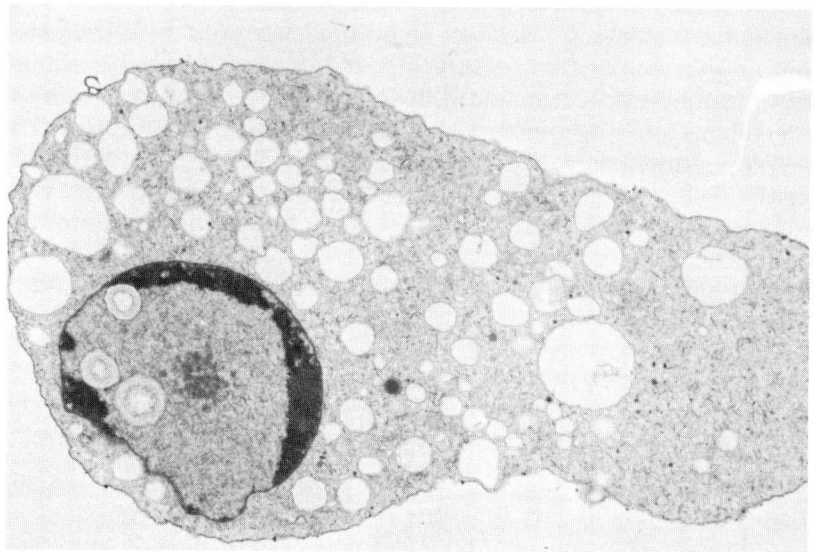

Figure 8. The cytoplasmic vesicles of trophozoites cultured in axenic media usually appear empty in thin sections. X 2,500.

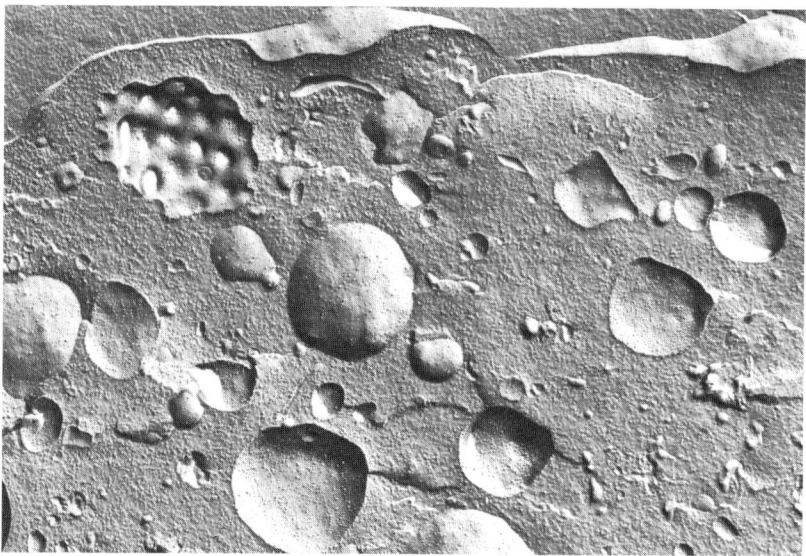

Figure 9. A freeze-fracture replica shows the presence of two populations of cytoplasmic vacuoles. X 8,000.

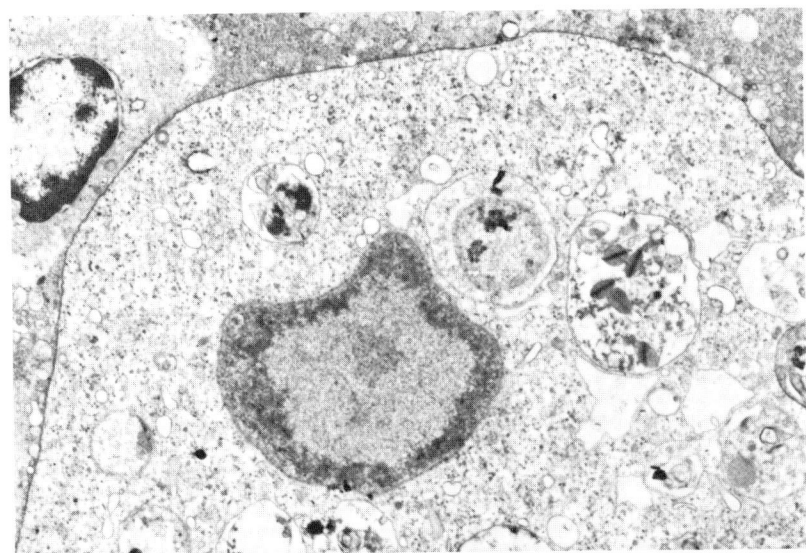

Figure 10. The cytoplasmic vacuoles of trophozoites obtained from liver lesions contain large amounts of cellular debris. X 4,000.

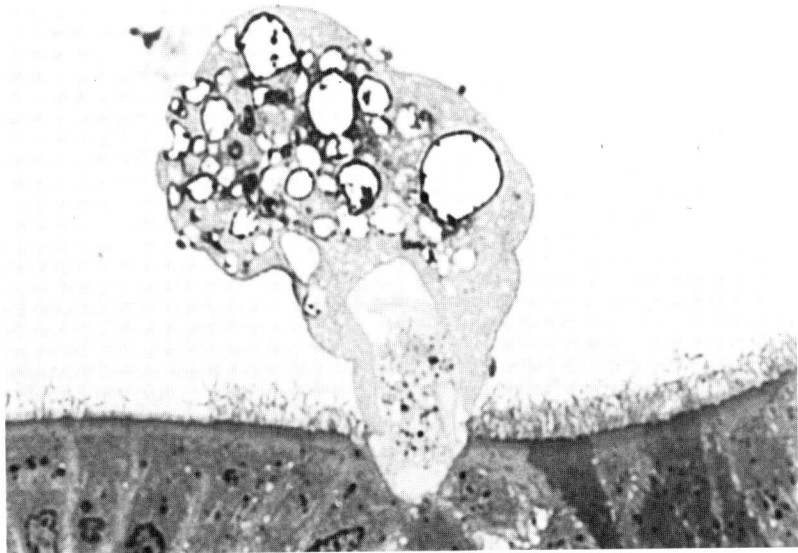

Figure 11. Light micrograph of a trophozoite adhered to the mucosal surface of the guinea pig cecum. Acid phosphatase-positive vacuoles are abundant. (Courtesy of Juan Mora Galindo.) X 1,800.

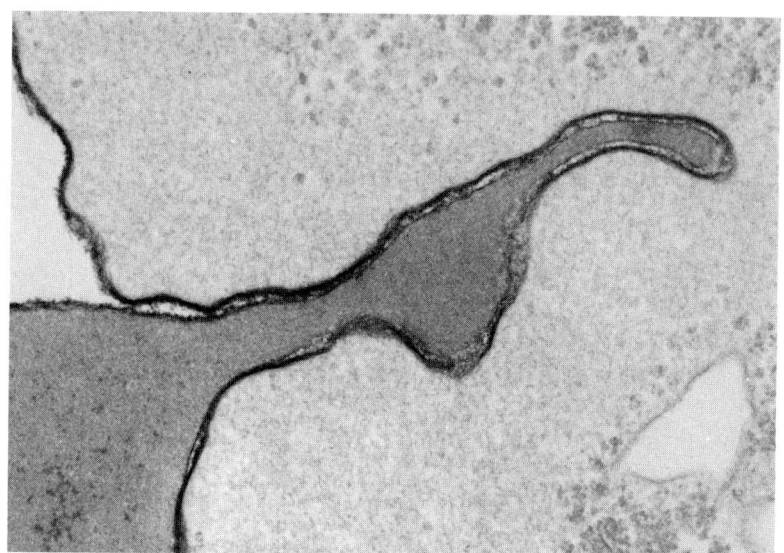

Figure 12. Phagocytosis of a red blood cells by a trophozoite. The shape of the red blood cell is distorted during ingestion. X 90,000.

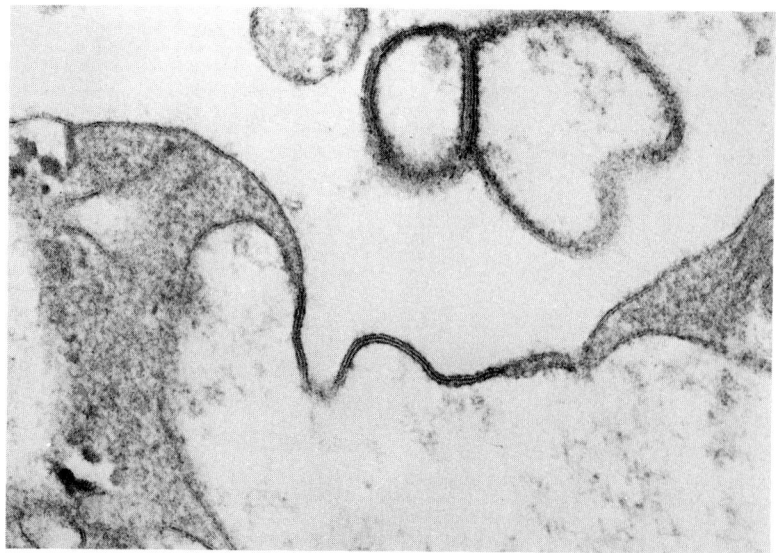

Figure 13. The rapid turnover of cytoplasmic vacuoles gives rise to many regions of membrane fusion between adjacent vacuoles, that appear as pentalaminar membranes. X 90,000.

The general configuration of the cytoplasmic vacuoles can be studied in freeze-fracture replicas of *E. histolytica*. Two populations can be defined on the basis of their surface features (Figure 9): the most abundant ones have a smooth contour, while the others appear to be crenated, since their surfaces are dotted with small bumps (Martínez-Palomo et al. 1976a). The significance of these morphological differences is not known. The phagocytic vacuoles of *E. histolytica* have been isolated by Kairalla et al (1976) after feeding trophozoites with 1–μm polystyrene latex beads. Initial attempts to explore the process of ingestion, digestion and liberation of degraded material by *E. histolytica* have involved the ultrastructural study of the phagocytic process in mammalian red blood cells (Treviño-García Manzo et al. 1971), cultured epithelial cells (McCaul 1977), and protozoa (Westphal and Michel 1971). The attachment of foreign particles to the surface of the amebas, their ingestion through phagocytic channels lined by ectoplasmic components, probably microfilaments, (Figure 12) and the various stages of cell degradation inside the vacuoles of *E. histolytica* have been described. However, there is little evidence relating the formation and subsequent internalization of phagocytic vacuoles with the fusion of lysosomal vesicles to initiate the degradation of the ingested material. Lushbaugh et al (1976) have suggested that images of membrane fusion are more frequent in freeze-fracture replicas of samples fixed by rapid freezing. Nevertheless, in actively phagocytic amebas, the fusion of membranes between adjacent phagocytic vacuoles can be found (Figure 13). Probably the most convincing evidence for the fusion of cytoplasmic vacuoles following endocytosis and the formation of a reticular channel system has been obtained with the aid of the microcinematographic analysis of living amebas engaged in phagocytosis and pinocytosis (Chévez et al.1976).

2.2.2 Tubular system

Even though there is no doubt that cytoplasmic components similar to the rough endoplasmic reticulum and the Golgi system, characteristic of protein-exporting eukaryotic cells, are lacking in the cytoplasm of *E. histolytica*, Ludvík and Shipstone (1970) have noted the existence of a membranous reticulum composed of fine tubules. This system has been interpreted as the counterpart of the typical smooth endoplasmic reticulum; i.e., a system of branching tubular elements constituting a compact three-dimensional lattice whose membrane surfaces are devoid of ribosomes. In fact, a lattice of tubules and vesicles superficially resembling smooth endoplasmic

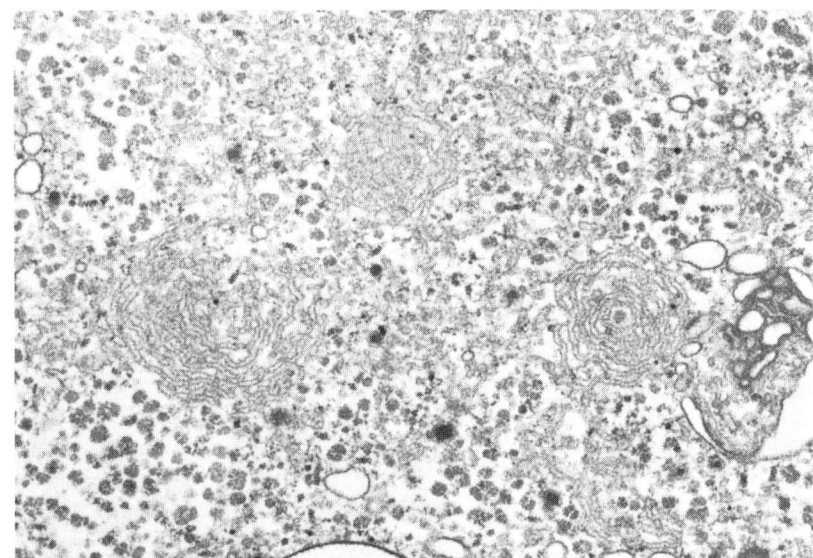

Figure 14. Irregular arrays of membrane-bound tubules are occasionally seen in the cytoplasm of trophozoites. X 12,500.

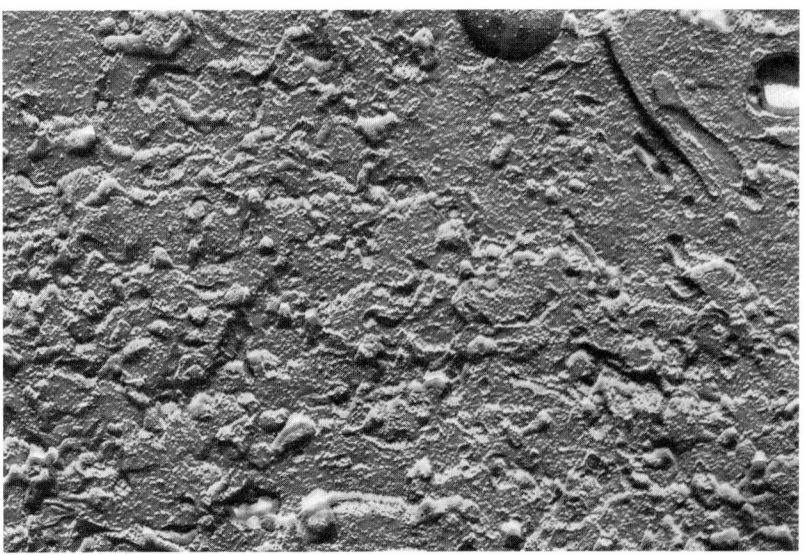

Figure 15. Freeze-fracture replica of membrane-bound tubules, similar to those seen in thin section in Figure 14. X 12,500.

reticulum can infrequently be found in the cytoplasm of *E. histolytica*, both in thin sections or in freeze-fracture replicas (Figures 14 and 15). When present, the system is made up of extremely thin tubules of approximately 20 nm in diameter, forming irregular whorls or parallel arrays. While the membrane of the vacuolar system in the trophozoites resembles the plasma membrane, both being approximately 10 nm thick, the membrane enclosing the tubules is only 6 nm thick.

Certain amebic products are liberated into the extracellular environment, including toxins that damage target epithelial tissues and enzymes that facilitate the invasion of solid tissues by the parasite. Whether these substances are channeled by means of membrane-bound compartments through the cell surface or whether they remain attached to the membrane components has yet to be determined.

At present, even though the cytoplasmic organization of *E. histolytica* is simple, it is not possible to separate those membrane components involved in the internalization and degradation of external components from those related to the synthesis, channeling, concentration, packaging, and liberation of extracellular products.

2.2.3 Ribosomal helical arrays

Free ribosomes are difficult to identify in thin sections of *E. histolytica* with the electron microscope. In growing cultured trophozoites and in amebas obtained from intestinal lesions, many ribosomes appear to be ordered in helical arrays approximately 300 nm in length and 40 nm in diameter (Figures 16–19). The individual elements of the helical arrays are 20–25 nm in diameter. In cysts and resting cultured trophozoites, the helices aggregate in large crystalline inclusions that are up to several micrometers in length, constituting the classical "chromatoid body" (Dobell 1919), seen with the light microscope. Under the electron microscope, chromatoid bodies appear as ordered helical arrays following a clear-cut hexagonal pattern (Figure 17). Barker and Deutsch (1958) found by histochemical tests that the chromatoid body of *E. invadens* is mainly composed of ribonucleoprotein, and demonstrated with the electron microscope that the crystals are made up of aggregated dense cytoplasmic particles. Further studies on the ultrastructure of the chromatoid bodies in *E. invadens* were carried out by Siddiqui and Rudzinska (1965). Ultraviolet absorption studies (Barker and Svihla 1964) and preliminary sedimentation analysis together with electron microscopic studies (Morgan et al. 1968) suggested that the chromatoid body is made up of ribosomes or ribosomal precursors. In fact, the three-dimensional reconstruction of electron micrographs has demonstrated that the asymmetrical unit of the ribonucleoprotein helix in *E. invadens* is composed of three particles; two of them probably are the large and small subunits of typical eukaryotic ribosomes, while the significance of the third remains unknown (Lake and Slayter 1972). The structure of the ribosomal helices in trophozoites and in the chromatoid bodies of cysts appears to be similar, as shown by electron microscopy and optical diffraction studies (Barker and Swales 1972b). Biochemical studies of helices isolated from trophozoites and cysts have given conflicting results; Kusamrarn et al (1975b) suggest that they are identical to ribosomes, while Barker and Swales (1972a) found that ribosomes from growing trophozoites of *E. invadens* have sedimentation velocities characteristic of eukaryotes (i.e., monomers average 80S; large subunits, 60S; and small subunits, 40S), while those obtained from cyst ribonucleoprotein crystals have higher sedimentation velocities. Although there is some evidence for extraribosomal components in chromatoid bodies (Kress et al.1971; Czeto et al.1973), no indisputable biochemical evidence of their existence has been found.

The nature of chromatoid bodies has mainly been explored in *E. invadens,* since this species is easier to culture and grows at room temperature, and, in addition, rapid and effective encystation can be experimentally induced. The chromatoid bodies of *E. histolytica* are sensitive to RNAase treatment (Rosenbaum and Wittner 1970), and incorporate tritiated ^{3}H-uridine (Kress et al. 1971). Furthermore, we have found that their constituent helices give a positive reaction using Bernhard's selective cytochemical technique for the ultrastructural detection of RNA-containing components (Figure 20). In *E. histolytica* trophozoites, helices are frequently found in association with digestive vacuoles (Rosenbaum and Wittner 1970), and in some sections a large number of helices are associated with membranous cisternae (Figure 19). In trophozoites grown in monophasic medium, Kress et al. (1971) found that the helix is the main form of ribosomal organization, whereas large chromatoid bodies appear in biphasic medium. These authors reported that ribonucleoprotein crystals can be induced in trophozoites by treatment with vinblastine.

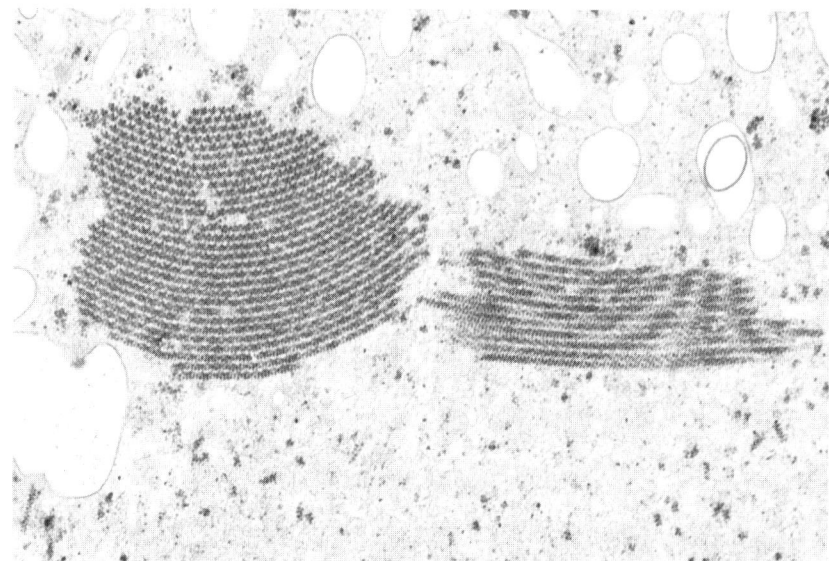

Figure 16. Thin section of a chromatoid body showing helical arrays of ribosomes. X 12,500.

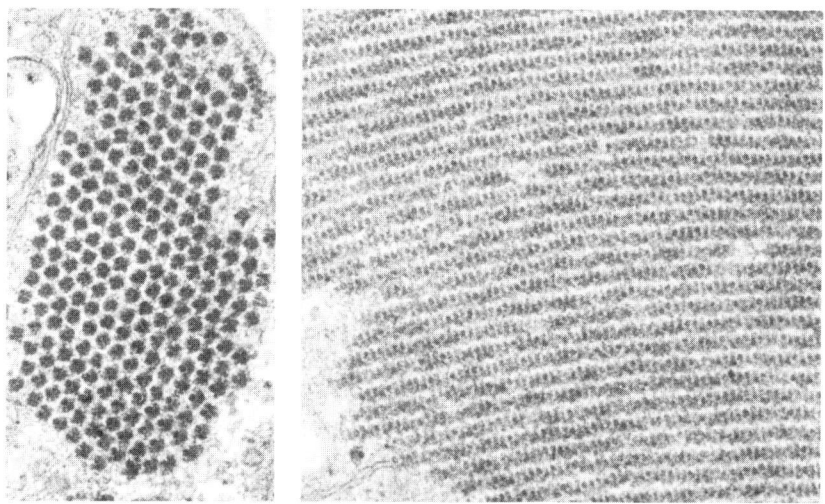

Figure 17. A transverse section through a chromatoid body reveals the hexagonal pattern of the helical arrays. X 54,000.

Figure 18. Parallel section of a chromatoid body that shows the disposition of individual particles. X 50,000.

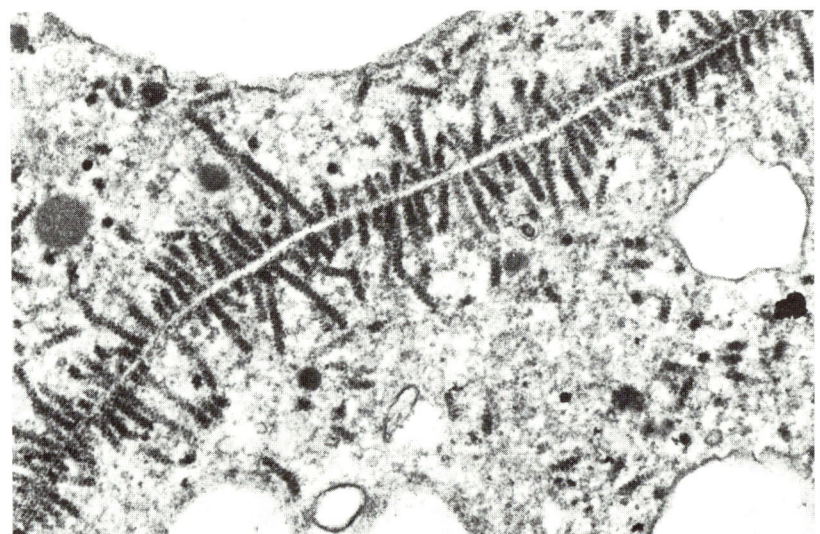

Figure 19. Membrane-bound helical arrays of ribosomes. X 25,000.

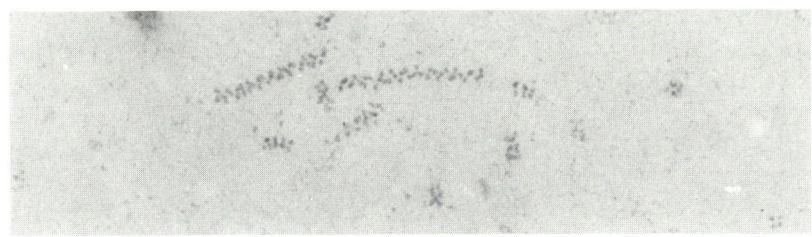

Figure 20. The helical arrays of ribosomes give a positive reaction using the cytochemical technique devised by Bernhard for the selective staining of RNA-containing components. X 50,000.

The functional significance of helical ribosomal arrays in *Entamoeba* remains an unsettled issue. According to Barker and Swales (1972a), the helices are formed by immature precursor particles synthesized during encystation. They suggest that, analogous with certain vertebrate oocytes and embryos, great numbers of ribosomes are synthesized which are not utilized until suitable conditions for growth and differentiation occur, and therefore, the particles or "ribosomogens" (Barker and Swales 1972a) could be ribosomal precursors with a different sedimentation value than that of normal active ribosomal monomers. These authors consider the formation of chromatoid bodies to be an essential step in preparation for differentiation. On the other hand, Kusamrarn et al (1975a) assume that aggregation occurs whenever ribosomes are unable to participate in the translation cycle, and thus agree with the classical view that the formation of chromatoid bodies is related with periods of reduced metabolic activity. These authors have demonstrated that chromatoid bodies can be induced in actively growing *E. invadens* trophozoites by treatment with various direct or indirect inhibitors of protein synthesis, and concluded that aggregates are composed of mature, normally functional ribosomes rendered free and inactive by a reduction in protein synthesis.

Chromatoid bodies in *Entamoeba* are one of the few available ordered systems of ribosomes ideally suited for use in three-dimensional studies, and as such have raised considerable interest among molecular biologists who are attempting to elucidate the relationship between structure and function in ribosomes of eukaryotic cells. Although helical ribosomal arrays have been described in a variety of vertebrate cell types and have been considered to be polyribosomes in some instances, their mode of formation and function remains obscure. It appears that members of the genus *Entamoeba* are the only cell types which normally have ribonucleoprotein helices as the major form of ribosomal organization in the cytoplasm. Isolation of intact helical arrays and the in vitro induction of crystal formation would greatly facilitate detailed biochemical analysis and probably permit x-ray diffraction analysis, which has not yet carried out (Morgan et al. 1968). When completed, these studies will reveal whether ribosomes in helices and in chromatoid bodies are functionally mature ribosomes or ribosomal precursors; furthermore, it is to be expected that they will greatly increase our knowledge of the structural organization of ribosomes in eukaryotic cells.

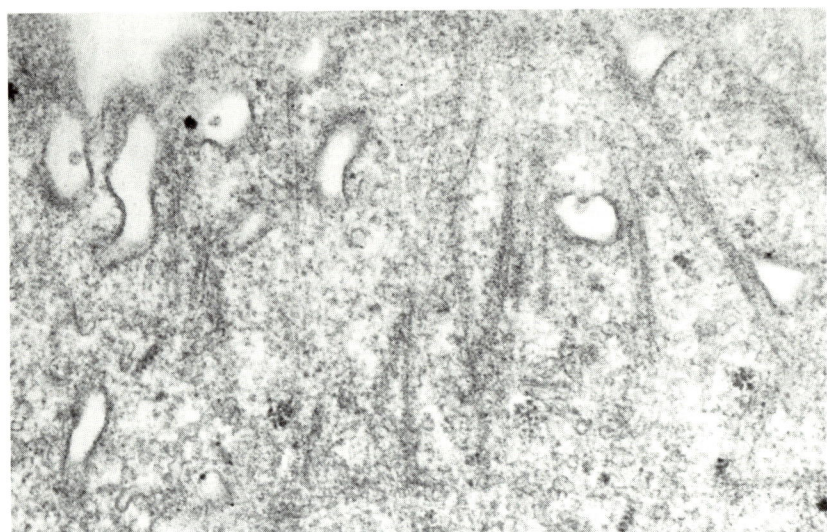

Figure 21. Microfilaments can be identified immediately beneath the plasma membrane at sites of attachment to the substrate. X 50,000.

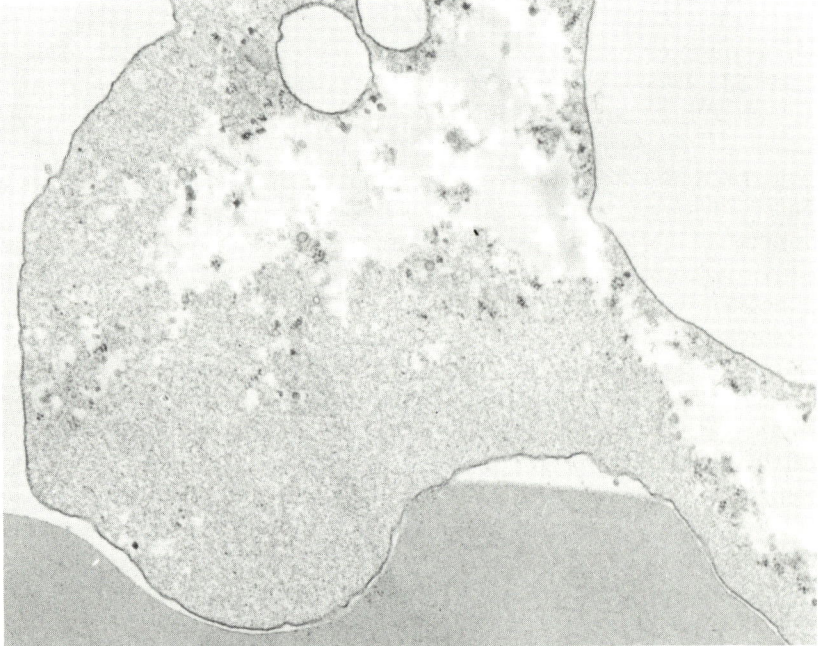

Figure 22. An ectoplasmic layer of fibrogranular material visible in phagocytic channels. Filaments have not been conclusively identified. X 90,000.

2.2.4 Cytoskeleton

During recent years, the cytoskeleton of nonmuscular cells has been a subject of considerable interest. At the ultrastructural level the cytoskeleton is composed of three different types of cytoplasmic fibrillar components involved in cellular movement and support: microfilaments made of actin, with an average diameter of 6-8 nm; tubulin-containing microtubules, 20-25 nm in diameter; and intermediate filaments, 10 nm thick. Despite the voluminous literature on the ultrastructure of *E. histolytica* trophozoites and the striking motility and plasticity of this protozoan, very little is known concerning the structural organization and biochemical characteristics of its cytoskeleton.

Even though microfilaments and microtubules are considered to be universal components of eukaryotic cells, there is only clear-cut evidence of the former in *E. histolytica*. In contrast, free-living amebas, such as *Acanthamoeba castellanii*, are excellent systems in which to study the structural and biochemical basis of contractility in nonmuscular cells. In addition to actin, present in high concentrations, these amebas have smaller amounts of a low molecular weight myosin, a cofactor protein required for actin-activation of the ATPase of myosin, and other proteins that are associated with actin (Korn 1975). *Acanthamoeba castellanii* trophozoites also have cytoplasmic microtubules (Bowers and Korn 1968).

Microfilaments have been identified with the electron microscope in the cytoplasm of *E. histolytica* trophozoites fixed in situ at growth temperature (Martínez-Palomo et al. 1974; Michel and Schupp 1975). They are short filaments approximately 7 nm in diameter, generally found immediately below the plasma membrane at the sites of attachment of the ameba to the substrate (Figure 21). Microfilaments are also found under the plasma membrane in regions where the cell surface is specialized to form phagocytic or macropinocytic channels (Figure 22). In these regions, a thick layer of fibrogranular material lines the inside of the endocytic invaginations. Once the endocytic channel is internalized, the corresponding vacuoles are no longer associated with the fibrogranular material. Definite fibrillar components are difficult to identify in the endocytic regions, even in specimens specially treated with low concentrations of osmium tetroxide and fixed at low temperature, conditions which are known to minimize microfilament depolymerization during fixation (Pollard and Maupin 1978). It would therefore seem that the microfilaments of *E. histolytica* involved in endocytic processes are particularly sensitive to fixation, probably because they are not associated with certain cytoskeletal proteins known to stabilize microfilaments in other eukaryotic cells. At any rate, microfilaments in trophozoites of *E. histolytica* do not appear to form well-defined bundles such as those present in vertebrate fibroblasts, since even in living motile trophozoites, no birefringent cytoplasmic components can be detected with polarization light microscopy. Several lines of evidence tend to support the notion that actin-containing microfilaments are present in *E. histolytica*: the presence of 7-nm filaments below the plasma membrane (Figure 21); the reduction of motility and intracellular movements of trophozoites after treatment with the drug cytochalasin B, that acts mainly through the depolymerization of microfilaments (Michel and Hohmann 1979); and the positive reaction to specific anti-actin antibodies in the cytoplasm of *E. histolytica* (Aust-Kettis et al. 1977). Thick filaments (9–14 nm in diameter) have been reported by Michel and Schupp (1975) but there is no proof that they are composed of myosin.

Microtubules similar to those found in almost all eukaryotic cells are not evident in thin sections of *E. histolytica* trophozoites. In well-characterized strains of *E. histolytica*, microtubules are absent in both the cytoplasm and nucleus of nondividing amebas. However, various investigators have reported the presence of microtubule-like structures in *E. histolytica*. Randomly oriented, electron-opaque microtubular structures, approximately 36 nm in diameter, have been described by Rosenbaum and Wittner (1970). Similar structures were reported in trophozoites by Michel and Schupp (1975) who found, in addition, that the components of these tubular structures may have a helical distribution. Neither the diameter nor the general ultrastructure of these components are characteristic of microtubules; they are present only exceptionally in the cytoplasm of *E. histolytica* and bear more of resemblance to reoviruses or unidentified filamentous viruses. As far as we know, there is no unambiguous biochemical or morphological identification of microtubules in the cytoplasm of *E. histolytica*; this is supported by the lack of activity of colchicine and related drugs that act on sensitive cells by inducing depolymerization of microtubules. Recent electron microscopic studies have shown microtubular bundles in the nuclei of dividing amebas of the genus *Entamoeba* (Gicquaud 1979; Injeyan et al. 1979). However, these observations pertain exclusively to *E. histolytica*-like Laredo type amebas. Keller et al. (1973) obtained indirect biochemical evidence suggesting the presence of tubulin in cysts of *E. invadens*, and mentioned the possible participation of tubulin-containing structures in the formation of chromatoid bodies. We have secured evidence of the presence of microtubular bundles in dividing nuclei of various pathogenic strains of *E. histolytica* (strains HM1:IMSS, HM38:IMSS, and HK9). In addition, we have found microtubular bundles in dividing trophozoites of *E. moshkovskii* and of certain isolates of *E. histolytica* obtained from cyst-passers.

Further studies on the cytoskeleton of *E. histolytica* are needed for a number of reasons. Trophozoites of *E. histolytica* provide an excellent model for the study of cytoskeleton-dependent phenomena such as endocytosis, and particularly, phagocytosis. In addition, motile processes are involved in certain phases of the cytopathic effect of virulent strains, such as adhesion, phagocytosis, and possibly, the export of toxic substances through exocytosis.

2.2.5 Cylindrical bodies

One of the characteristic cytoplasmic components of *E. histolytica* trophozoites, whether originating from cultures or from human intestinal or liver lesions, are the dense cylindrical particles, generally arranged bidimensionally as a rosette (Figure 23). These bodies were simultaneously described in trophozoites obtained from colonic exudates in cases of acute amebic colitis (El-Hashimi and Pittman 1970), hamster liver lesions (Lowe and Maegraith 1970c), and in axenic (Lowe and Maegraith 1970b; Treviño-García Manzo et al. 1970) and polyxenic (Lowe and Maegraith 1970a; Ludvík and Shipstone 1970) cultures. A more detailed description of the ultrastructure of these dense cylindrical bodies was given by Feria-Velasco and Treviño (1972). One or two rosette-like conglomerates of cylindrical particles are usually found in thin sections surrounding a finely granular specialized area of the cytoplasm (Figure 23). These conglomerates measure about 1 μm in diameter and are composed of 9–30 cylindrical bodies. The bodies vary in size up to 250 nm in length and 90 nm in diameter, and are limited by a membrane approximately 7 nm thick (Figure 24). They tend to be bullet-shaped in appearance, flat at one end and in the form of a tapered sphere (Figure 24) at the other, although occasionally they appear rounded at both ends. The particles generally are organized in spherical arrays that in sections give the appearance of a rosette; however, isolated particles can also be found, usually in association with cytoplasmic vacuoles or the cell periphery.

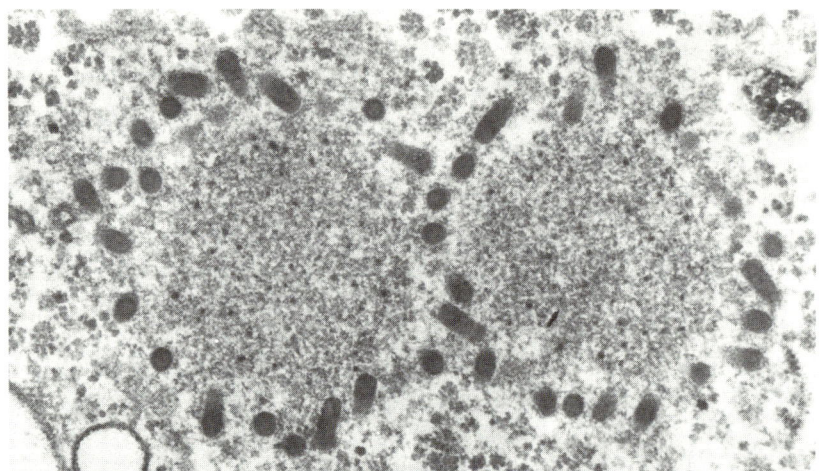

Figure 23. Rhabdovirus-like particles from two rosettes. X 40,000.

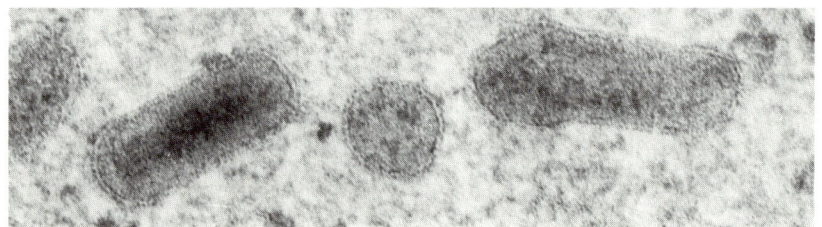

Figure 24. High magnification of several rhabdovirus-like particles. X 150,000.

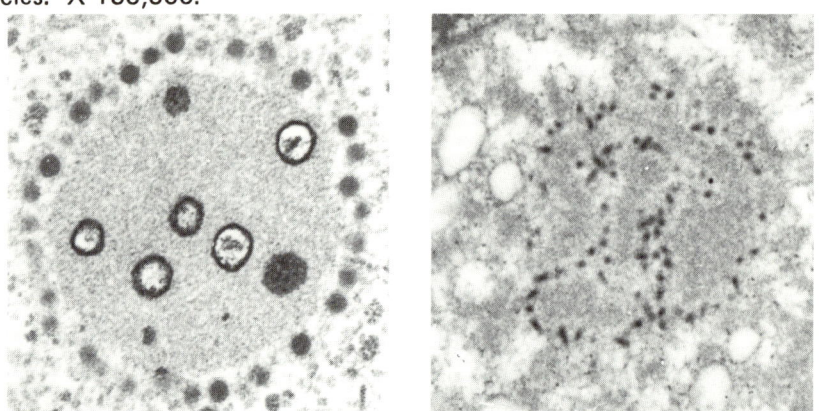

Figure 25. "Nuclear" inclusions in a rosette. X 30,000.
Figure 26. Particles are positive to Bernhard's RNA technique. X 20,000.

Rosette arrangements of cylindrical bodies are particularly prominent in trophozoites of *E. histolytica* obtained from human amebic liver abscesses, and are absent in the cytoplasm of the nonpathogenic *Entamoeba coli* (Proctor 1976; Rondanelli et al.1977) and *Entamoeba gingivalis* (Rondanelli et al.1977). This observation and the resemblance of the particles to rhabdoviruses (Bird and McCaul 1976) have generated considerable interest in these components in view of their possible pathogenic role. Mattern et al (1976) have found that cylindrical particles differentiate into "T-bars" in amebas that are undergoing degeneration either spontaneously or following viral infection. According to this investigator, the appearance of the particles suggests a bacteriophage-like entity with the capacity to escape from dying cells and reinfect apparently normal amebas. He further emphasized that the presence of "nuclear inclusions" in some rosettes (Figure 25) is compatible with the nuclear origin of the material incorporated into the cylindrical particles.

Bird and McCaul (1976) found cylindrical particles in the cytoplasm of trophozoites of twelve different pathogenic strains of *E. histolytica*, including a Laredo strain, and in a strain of *E. invadens*. On the basis of the structural similarity with well-characterized rhabdoviruses, Bird and McCaul (1976) suggest that the particles are RNA rhabdoviruses, and speculate on the possible involvement of such putative viruses in the transfer of genetic markers, including virulence factors, between bacteria and trophozoites.

At present, it is not possible to make a definite statement concerning the nature of the cylindrical bodies found in *E. histolytica*. They resemble rhabdoviruses in a number of morphological features that include:

a) Size. Rhabdoviruses are rod-shaped particles varying considerably in length, from 60 to 400 nm, but of consistent width, 60–85 nm (Wagner 1975).

b) Shape. Animal rhabdoviruses tend to be bullet-shaped in appearance, while plant rhabdoviruses have two rounded ends.

c) Presence of a membranous envelope in both cylindrical particles and rhabdoviruses.

d) Existence of a dense RNA-containing core, shown with the selective cytochemical technique for RNA detection in water-soluble sections (Figure 26), described by Bernhard.

e) Morphological similarity between the specialized granular area inside the rosette arrangement of cylindrical particles and the cytoplasmic foci of rhabdovirus synthesis (Hummeler and Tomassini 1973).

f) Evidence of a helical arrangement of the inner contents of the cylindrical particles (Bird and McCaul 1976) that resemble the ribonucleocapsid core of rhabdoviruses which have a striated appearance when viewed with the electron microscope (Wagner 1975).

On the other hand, certain features of the cylindrical particles are not consistent with their viral nature, for example:

a) Efforts to infect experimental animals or to establish viral replication in cultured cells have failed (Bird and McCaul 1976).

b) Cylindrical particles do not show the characteristic surface spikes that correspond to the so-called G protein of rhabdovirus envelopes, involved in the attachment of the virion to the membranes of host cells.

c) Electron microscopy of cylindrical particles in amebas has not revealed intermediate stages similar to those found during the cycle of infection of cultured cells with rhabdoviruses, such as the entry of mature particles or the budding of infective virions.

d) The cylindrical particles are always found in very small numbers.

Rhabdoviruses are ubiquitous, highly infectious agents of animal and plant diseases, and therefore their possible presence in a pathogenic protozoan is not unlikely. However, even if the cylindrical particles found in the cytoplasm of *E. histolytica* trophozoites are eventually proved to be rhabdoviruses, their presumptive role as vehicles for the transfer of virulence factors has yet to be demonstrated.

2.2.6 Filamentous and polyhedral viruses

E. histolytica cultures contain viruses that become evident when the amebal lysate of a given strain is incubated with a culture of a sensitive strain (Diamond et al. 1972). As a result, two morphological types of DNA viruses are produced by the infected cultures: a filamentous virus and a polyhedral virus, detectable by electron microscopy (Mattern et al.1972; Hruska et al.1973). These viral particles are not observed in healthy axenic cultures (Diamond and Mattern 1976). The viruses are probably integrated into amebal genomes in a classic lysogenic system. Diamond and Mattern (1976) have been unable to infect animals, bacterial cultures, or cultured mammalian cells with these viruses. Although the possibility that the virulence of amebas could be related to the presence of viruses is of much interest, no evidence has been obtained for such a relationship, as has been found in the case of the lysogenic conversion of nontoxigenic to toxigenic bacterial strains (Mattern et al.1979).

2.3 The Cell Surface

The plasma membrane of *E. histolytica* is approximately 10 nm thick and shows the classical unit membrane appearance of biological membranes in perpendicular sections (Figure 27). This membrane is thicker than the plasma membranes of mammalian cells, most of which measure approximately 8 nm. The plasma membrane of cultured *E. histolytica* trophozoites is covered on the outer face by a barely detectable surface coat (Figure 28), demonstrable with the use of cytochemical reagents that enhance the electron density of carbohydrate-containing membrane components, such as ruthenium red or alcian blue (Lushbaugh and Miller 1974; Pinto da Silva et al. 1975). The surface coat is of particular interest because it probably contains some of the amebic antigens recognized as foreign by the host during the establishment of invasive amebiasis. In addition, the pathogenic action of the amebas may depend upon direct contact with host cells, and the virulence of the amebas may thus be related to the composition and properties of the surface coat components.

2.3.1 The surface coat

When ruthenium red or alcian blue are used together with osmium tetroxide, the surface coat of *E. histolytica* appears to be formed by short filaments, 6–10 nm in length, uniformly distributed over the cell surface. The surface coat may contain exposed mannose or glucose residues, since it binds the lectin concanavalin A which interacts specifically with those sugars (Martínez-Palomo et al. 1973). The binding of this lectin has been demonstrated in *E. histolytica* with the aid of the peroxidase technique devised by Bernhard and Avrameas (1971).

As a result of the interaction with specific ligands, surface coat components accumulate at the uroid and are later eliminated into the medium. Even in the absence of specific ligands, a continuous shedding of surface components appears to take place in actively moving trophozoites of *E. histolytica*. As the cells move along, a thin layer of material is deposited on the substrate, where it accumulates as a microexudate with cytochemical properties similar to those of the surface coat of trophozoites (Figure 29) (Pinto da Silva and Martínez-Palomo 1974; Pinto da Silva et al. 1975). This shedding mechanism of surface components may also be of interest when evaluating the means of evasion of the immune response.

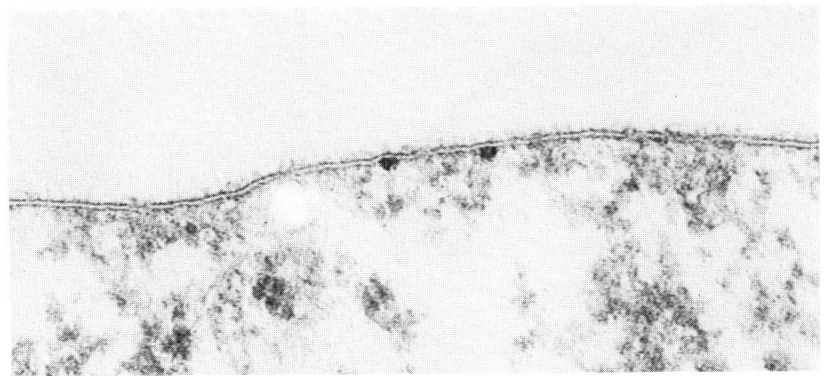

Figure 27. In cross section the plasma membrane of trophozoites show a trilaminar structure. X 100,000.

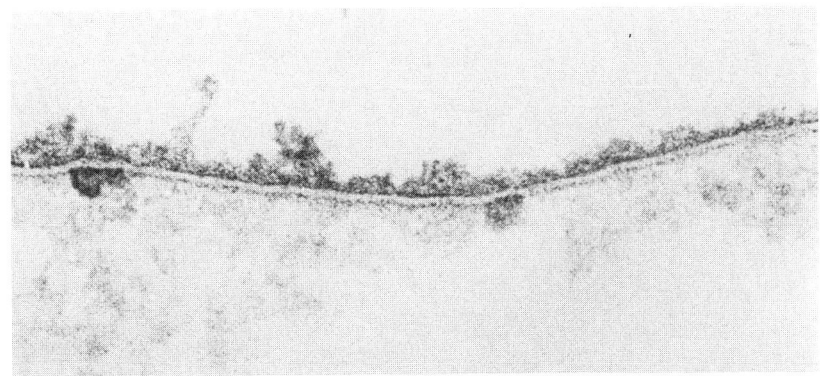

Figure 28. The plasma membrane is covered by a thin and irregular surface coat detectable with ruthenium red. X 120,000.

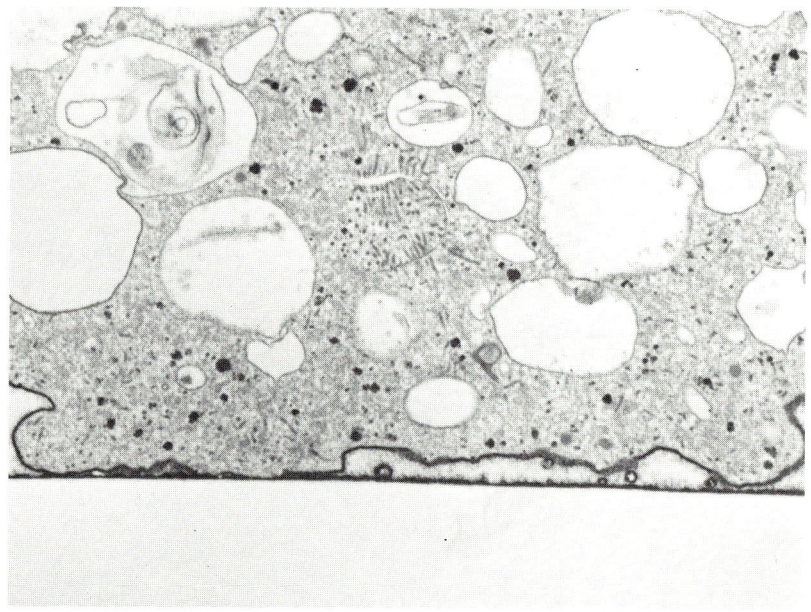

Figure 29. A thin layer of microexudate is deposited on the substrate as trophozoites move. X 10,000.

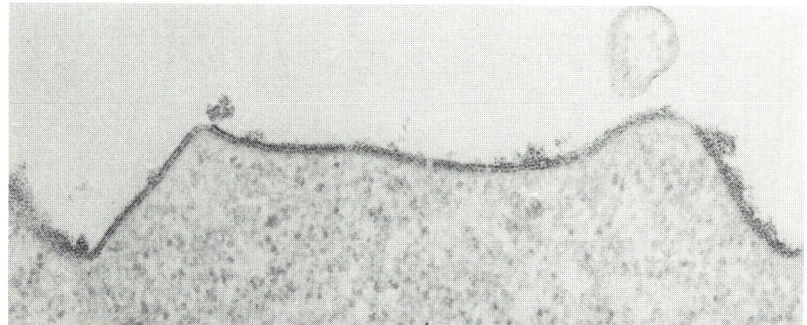

Figure 30. Heavy binding of cationic ferritin at the cell surface of an *E. histolytica*-like, Laredo type trophozoite. X 35,000.

Electron microscopic studies have shown variations in the thickness of the surface coat of *E. histolytica* trophozoites depending on the origin of the amebas. Surface coats have been reported to be more prominent in invasive forms of amebas obtained from colonic lesions (El-Hashimi and Pittman 1970) and from liver abscesses (Proctor 1976). According to Lushbaugh and Miller (1974), the surface coats of monoxenically cultured amebas taken from intestinal lesions are about twice as thick as those of axenic cells. We have corroborated this observations by measuring the thickness of the surface coat of amebas from the strain HM1:IMSS cultured under axenic or monoxenic conditions. The latter is approximately 12.8 nm thick, whereas the surface coat of axenic trophozoites of the same strain averages 10.0 nm. As detailed elsewhere, there is evidence that the components of the surface coat are loosely bound to the cell surface and therefore can be washed off easily during the preparative procedures for electron microscopy. In addition, the surface of *E. histolytica* may bind serum components that would add to the thickness of the surface coat. Therefore, differences between the surface coats of amebas obtained from various sources should be interpreted with caution (Martínez-Palomo et al.1980b).

The surface coats of certain strains of *E. histolytica* of low virulence can be labeled with cationic ferritin at neutral pH, as revealed by electron microscopy (Figure 30). These strains have an overall negative electrical charge at the cell surface, demonstrable by microelectrophoresis. However, virulent strains of *E. histolytica* do not have measurable electrophoretic mobility at neutral pH and do not bind cationic ferritin under these conditions (Trissl et al. 1977). The chemical basis for this difference in the electrokinetic properties of virulent and nonvirulent amebas is not known.

Most eukaryotic cells contain sialic acid (neuraminic acid) as one of the significant components of the surface coat. This carbohydrate appears to be absent from the surface of *E. histolytica*, since colloidal iron binding at low pH is not modified by previous incubation with neuraminidase. Furthermore, direct chemical analysis of the surface components has failed to reveal the existence of sialic acid in *E. histolytica* (Feria-Velasco et al.1973).

2.3.2 The plasma membrane

The plasma membranes of motile forms of *E. histolytica* have been studied with the freeze-fracture method which permits the visualization of components located in the middle, or hydrophobic,

Figure 31. Freeze-fracture replica of the E face of the plasma membrane. Few membrane particles are seen. X 120,000.

Figure 32. Freeze-fracture replica of the P face of the plasma membrane. Membrane particles are numerous and heterogeneous. X 120,000.

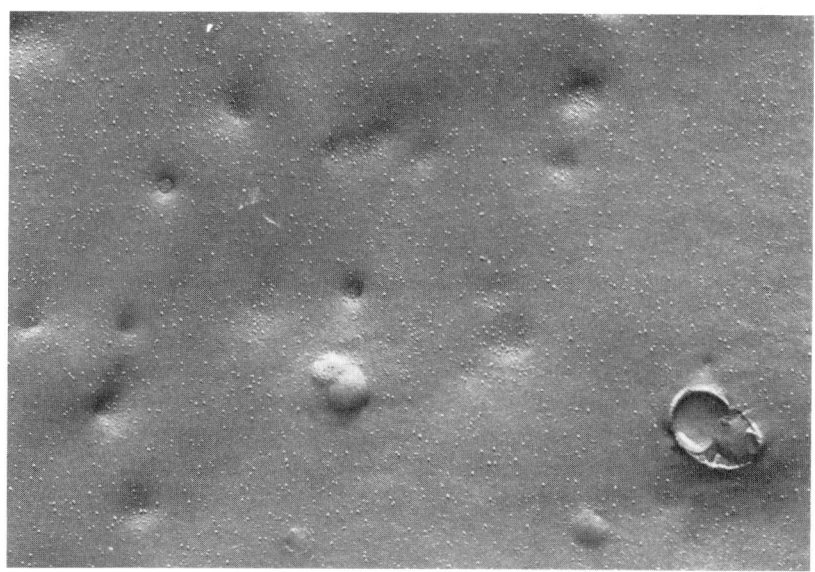

Figure 33. Freeze-fracture replica of the plasma membrane of a trophozoite (P face). Regions of exocytosis, micropinocitosis, and particle-enriched depressed regions are found. X 50,000.

region of the membrane. As in other eukaryotic cells, the inner half of the plasma membrane, or P face, that is in contact with the ectoplasm is covered by an abundant and heterogeneous population of membrane particles, most of which appear to be integral proteins. In comparison, the complementary E face that occupies the external side of the plasma membrane has a less abundant population of membrane particles (Martínez-Palomo et al. 1976b) (Figures 31, 32). No specialized distribution of membrane particles has been found in *E. histolytica*; therefore, the regions containing micropinocytic channels and pseudopodia show no modifications in terms of the disposition of membrane particles. Linear arrangements of particles have been described (Martínez-Palomo et al. 1976b), but their significance is unknown. A remarkable feature of the freeze-fracture morphology of *E. histolytica* trophozoites is the presence of circumscribed areas of the membrane which display a much higher density of membrane particles. These flattened particle-enriched regions have an irregular contour and their largest dimension reaches 0.5 μm (Martínez-Palomo et al. 1976b). Images of membrane fusion between cytoplasmic vacuoles and the plasma membrane during exocytosis are frequently obtained in *E. histolytica*. Regions of endocytosis through micro- or macropinocytosis also lack a specialized distribution of membrane particles (Figure 33). It is likely that future advances in the knowledge of the chemical composition of membrane components of *E. histolytica* will render possible the identification of specific molecular species of proteins in terms of given populations of membrane particles seen by freeze-fracture, thus integrating morphological information concerning the protein components of the plasma membrane with the biochemical data.

2.3.3 Capping

A rapid polar redistribution of certain surface components of *E. histolytica* follows the interaction with a variety of external ligands such as lectins, polyspecific antibodies, and cationic ferritin (Figure 34). The normal distribution of receptors and antigens on the surface of amebas is uniform over the outer aspect of the cell, but at certain temperatures and ligand concentrations, the surface determinants move over the plasma membrane and accumulate at the posterior part, or uroid, of the cell (Pinto da Silva et al. 1975). Under optimal conditions, caps may be found in more than 70% of a given culture after interaction with a ligand (Trissl et al. 1978).

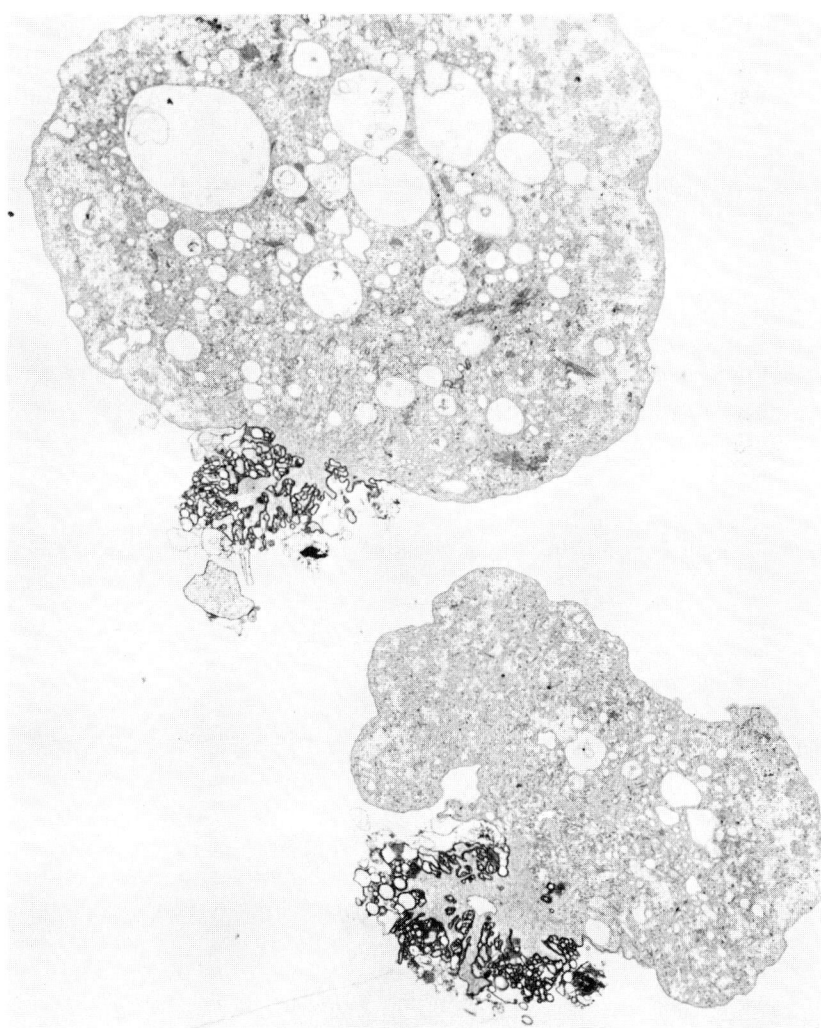

Figure 34. Caps are visible at the uroid of trophozoites incubated with concanavalin A and peroxidase before fixation. The lectin receptors are rapidly redistributed and concentrated at the posterior end of the amebas. X 3,000.

Our suggestion that the capping phenomenon could be a powerful mechanism for the removal of antibodies from the surface of *E. histolytica* was reinforced by the results of Aust-Kettis and Sundqvist (1978). However, these authors reported that a double layer of antibodies was needed in order to induce surface caps. Recently, Calderón et al (1980) induced capping of surface antigens with a single layer of antibodies against *E. histolytica* using higher concentrations of immunoglobulin. In contrast with the capping process in white blood cells, the surface segregation in *E. histolytica* is accompanied by extensive folding of the membrene at the caps, followed by the spontaneous release of the evaginated membrane region. It is feasible that both the surface redistribution of membrane antigens and the subsequent release of the cap through the contraction of a constriction ring are regulated by cytoskeletal components, mainly actin microfilaments that accumulate at the uroid region in capped amebas. The possibility that the rapid disappearance of antigen-antibody complexes from the parasite surface may render the ameba less susceptible to the humoral immune response is under study at present.

A rapid movement of surface molecules following interaction with a ligand has been reported in other protozoan parasites such as *Leishmania* (Doyle et al.1974), *Trypanosoma cruzi* (Schmuñis et al.1980), and *Trypanosoma brucei* (Barry 1979).

2.3.4 Shedding

The dynamic nature of the cell surface of *E. histolytica* is not only reflected in the swift mobilization of antibodies after binding to surface antigens through capping, but also in the constant release of surface molecules into the extracellular environment which could eventually interfere with the effective mediation of cellular immunity against invading protozoa. In thin sections of *E. histolytica* cultures that have been fixed, dehydrated, and embedded in situ (Martínez-Palomo et al.1974), amebas are found to deposit a thin layer of microexudate which is invariably attached to the substrate (Pinto da Silva et al.1975). The microexudate appears as a nearly uniform dense coat approximately 5 nm in thickness and shows cytochemical reactivity similar, but not identical, to that of the surface coat of trophozoites, suggesting that not all the components of the surface coat are exfoliated (Figure 29).

In addition to the deposition of a microexudate on the substrate, a pronounced shedding of surface components is induced by the incubation of living trophozoites with a high concentration of ligands (lectins or antibodies). Under these conditions, a certain proportion of cells form caps of ligand-receptor complexes, while a significant number of amebas liberate sheets of surface coat components containing receptors or antigens, revealed by immunofluorescence microscopy using fluorescein-tagged ligands.

The shedding process resembles the "exudation" of antigen-antibody complexes described in ciliated protozoa such as *Tetrahymena* and *Paramecium*. Biochemical labeling experiments carried out with *Acanthamoeba castellanii* have indicated that the surface coat material is in fact a precursor of the microexudate (Pigon 1978). In the case of *E. histolytica*, the nature of the microexudate is unknown, but the possibility that it contains soluble antigenic material warrants the study of the synthesis and turnover of membrane-associated antigens.

2.3.5 Dense oval bodies

The inner leaflet of the trilaminar plasma membrane of *E. histolytica* contains dense oval bodies which frequently can be observed in thin sections (Figure 27). They are irregular in size and shape, but average about 30 by 50 nm. First described by Rondanelli et al. (1965) in *E. invadens*, they were later found in cultured forms of *E. histolytica* (Rondanelli, 1966), *E. moshkovskii* (Ludvík and Shipstone 1970), and *E. coli* (Rondanelli et al. 1974), but have not been described in *E. histolytica* trophozoites obtained from human liver abscesses (Proctor 1976). An interesting feature of these bodies is that although they are mainly located in the plasma membrane, they are present in much lesser amounts in the inner cytoplasmic membranes despite the apparently rapid turnover between the outer and inner membranes. The nature of these bodies has been the subject of much speculation. They have been alternatively considered to be related to the cytopathic activity of *E. histolytica*, the contractile activity of the cell surface, the synthesis of cell membranes, or to represent "directional" chemotactic centers (Ludvík and Shipstone 1970). Therefore, although they have served to stimulate the imagination of electron microscopists, little more than their mere existence has been confirmed. Taking into account their morphology and constant relationship with the plasma membrane, the dense oval bodies can be likened to the Ca^{++}-binding sites demonstrated in various protozoa such as *Acanthamoeba* (Sobota et al 1978), *Tetrahymena*, and *Amoeba proteus*. In these cells, the Ca^{++}-binding membrane sites might constitute a Ca^{++} regulating system that could control the function of contractile microfilaments located around the periphery of the cell. Whether or not dense oval bodies represent cation binding structures could be determined with the use of x-ray dispersion analysis.

2.3.6 Surface specializations

Electron microscopic examination of adequately fixed specimens reveals various structural differentiations of a transient nature at the surface of *E. histolytica* trophozoites. These surface specializations are extremely sensitive to changes in temperature and osmolarity, and therefore are only evident in amebas fixed in situ at growth temperature. Direct fixation of motile trophozoites prevents the disappearance of these surface modifications and the assumption of a spherical shape characteristic of trophozoites subjected to cooling and centrifugation before fixation (Martínez-Palomo et al 1974).

Two general types of transient surface specializations may be found: evaginations (pseudopodia: lobopodia and filopodia, and the uroid), and invaginations (phagocytic and macropinocytic vacuoles, and micropinocytic vesicles). All these differentiations may be present at a given time on the surface of an ameba. While evaginations are related to cell motility and attachment, invaginations reflect the various endocytic processes whereby amebas incorporate liquid and particulate material into the cytoplasm.

Lobopodia (Figure 35) are finger-like ectoplasmic protrusions that have a hyaline appearance in living cells. Under the transmission electron microscope, no major differences between the cytoplasmic matrix of the lobopodia and the remaining cytoplasm is found, except for the lack of vesicles and large particles in the evaginations. Membrane-like elements situated between the ectoplasmic and endoplasmic regions of lobopodia have been described in *E. invadens* by Zaman (1972); however, no true membranous barrier is present between these regions in the amebic cytoplasm. When viewed with the scanning electron microscope, the surfaces of the lobopodia appear strikingly smooth (Figure 36), in comparison to the wrinkled contours of the rest of the cell surface. Even though lobopodia have a higher negative surface charge density than the rest of the cell in certain small free-living amebas such as *Naegleria gruberi*, no local modifications of the

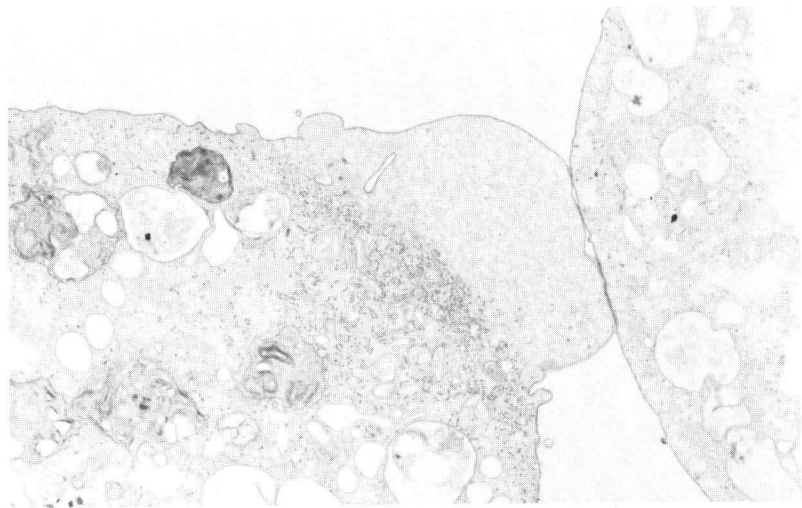

Figure 35. In thin sections lobopodia appear as ectoplasmic protrusions devoid of cytoplasmic vesicles. X 10,000.

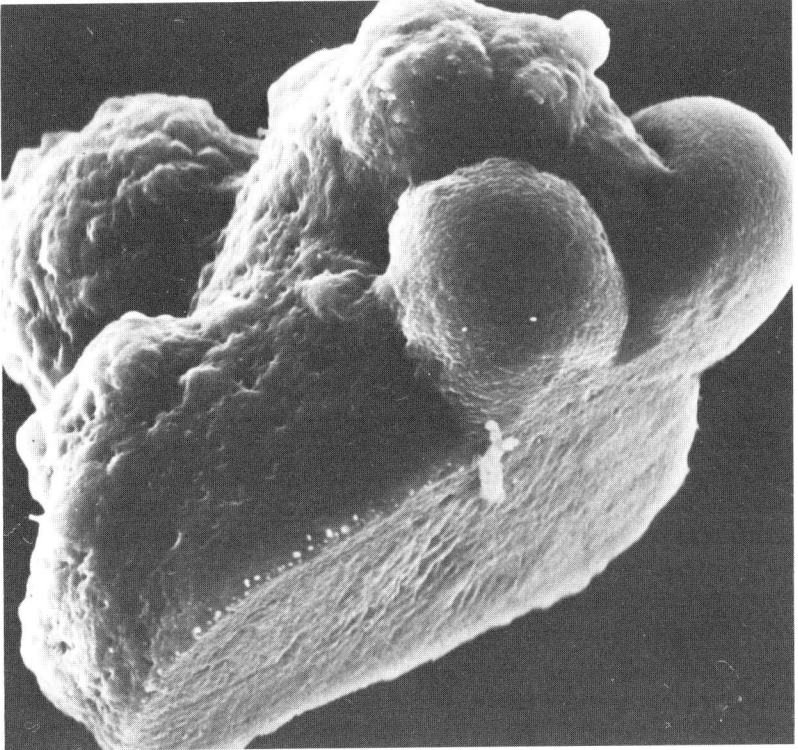

Figure 36. Scanning electron micrograph showing the smooth appearance of lobopodia surfaces. X 8,000.

surface coat can be detected with transmission electron microscopy in trophozoites of *E. histolytica* in which the surface coat components are revealed with ruthenium red, or the surface charge distribution is studied with cationic ferritin. Freeze-fracture electron microscopy reveals no modification of the disposition of intramembrane particles on the fractured faces of the plasma membrane during the explosive formation of pseudopodia.

In spite of the voluminous literature on the ultrastructure of motile forms of *E. histolytica*, filopodia remained undetected until recently. Improvements in fixation methods allowed the visualization of filopodia as long filiform extensions of the cell surface (Figure 37) (Martínez-Palomo et al 1974). The largest filopodia are associated with the uroid and are visible even with the light microscope (Hopkins and Warner 1946). Zaman (1972) illustrated the filopodia and termed them "long mucous threads." The difficulty in identifying filopodia with transmission electron microscopy stems not only from the fact that routine techniques for fixation are inadequate, but also because this particular form of pseudopodia is too long and irregular to be seen in its entirety in a single thin section. For these reasons, a detailed account of their ultrastructure was not given until serial sectioning followed by the three-dimensional reconstruction of consecutive images of filopodia profiles was carried out by Deas and Miller (1977). These authors described filopodia as "dendritic extensions" of the surface of amebas obtained from liver or colonic lesions. Lushbaugh and Pittman (1979) later applied other suitable ultrastructural techniques for the analysis of surface projections, such as high voltage transmission electron microscopy which permits the visualization of thick sections, and scanning electron microscopy of critical point-dried trophozoites (Figure 38) whose overall shape remains more or less intact. With these techniques, filopodia were seen in their entirety as filamentous surface projections extending several micrometers in length, occasionally reaching 100 μm, with a diameter of about 0.1 μm. The profiles of filopodia are irregular since bulbous swellings are present along their length. According to McCaul and Bird (1977), filopodia are present only on the basal side of trophozoites, although Lushbaugh and Pittman (1979) found them spread over the entire surface of the cell.

Since filopodia are far more prominent in trophozoites in contact with target epithelial cells, the possibility exists that these pseudopodia may be involved in attachment and/or cytopathic activity. In mammalian cells, the small dimensions of the tips of

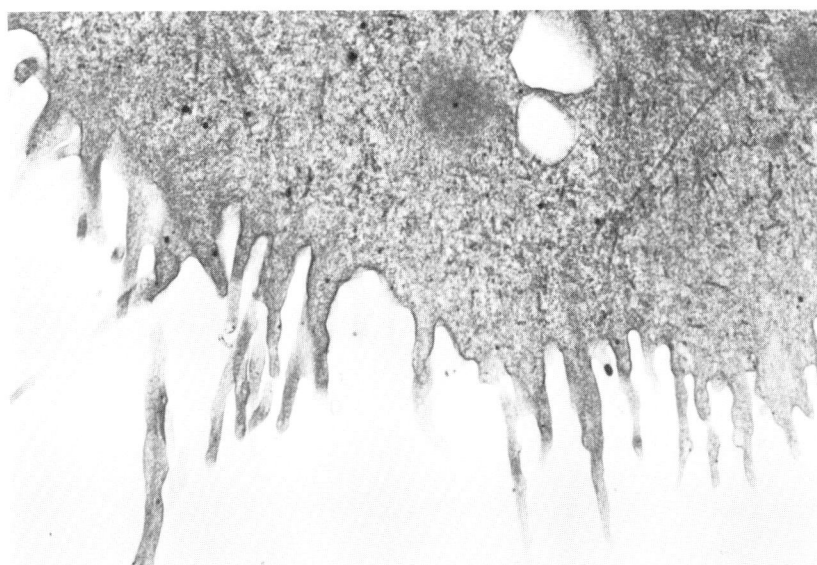

Figure 37. In favorable sections, filopodia may be seen on the periphery of the basal side of trophozoites in culture. X 16,000.

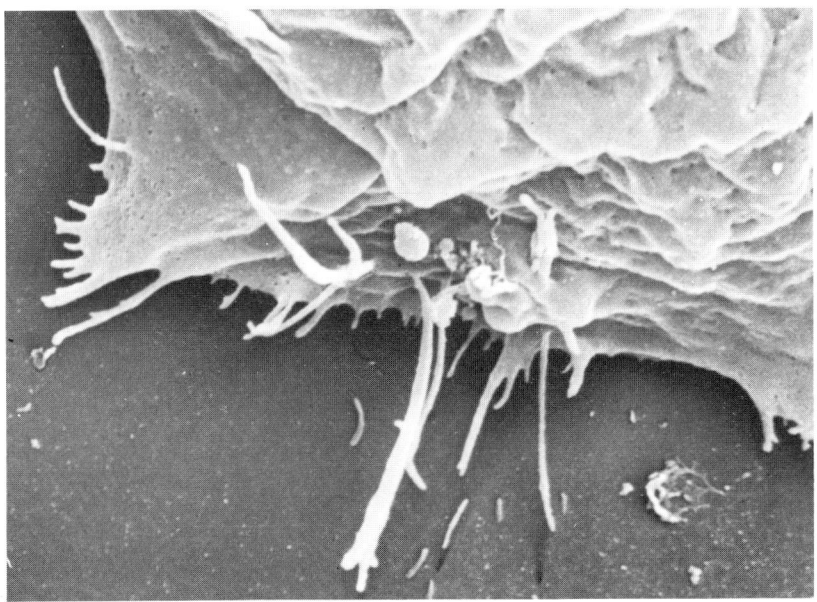

Figure 38. Filopodia are best evidenced in scanning electron micrographs of critical point-dried trophozoites. X 15,000.

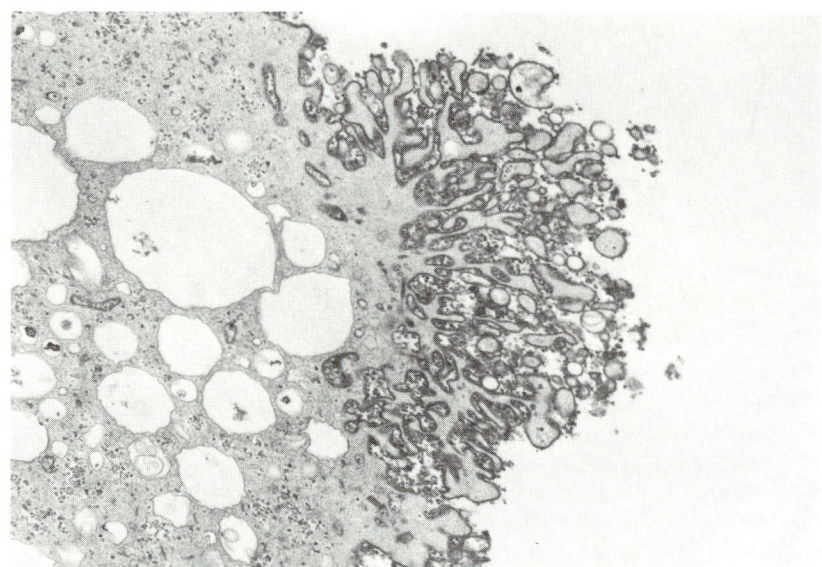

Figure 39. Uroid of a trophozoite incubated with cationic ferritin before fixation. X 10,000.

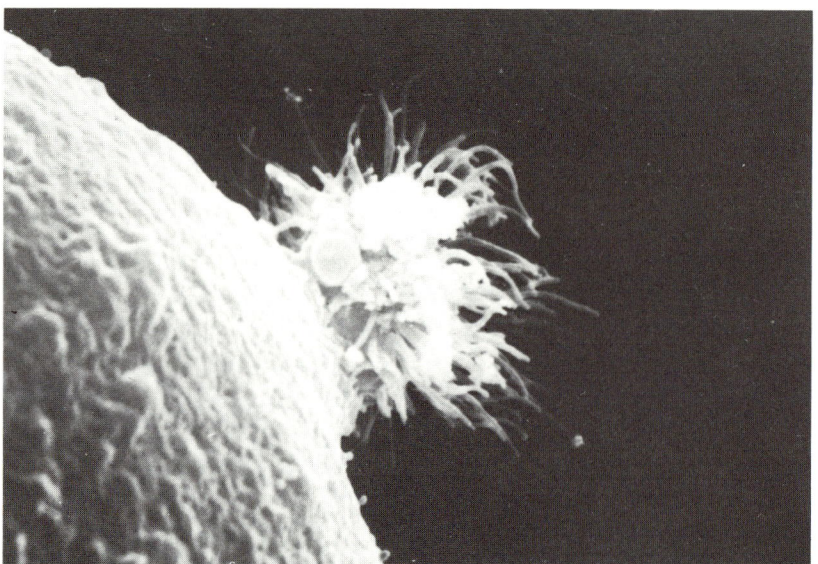

Figure 40. Uroid of a critical point-dried trophozoite visualized with the scanning electron microscope. X 8,000.

filopodia are thought to facilitate close interaction through the breakage of the physicochemical barriers of like repulsive forces between adjacent cells, thus bringing the cell membranes within a short distance of each other and making close contact possible (Rajaraman et al 1974). Deas and Miller (1977) suggest that filopodial membranes may contain cytotoxic hydrolases that act at the contact sites. McCaul and Bird (1977), in turn, assume that filopodia are mainly associated with cellular motility. Examination of large numbers of sections showing the interface between trophozoites and epithelial cells both in vitro and in vivo has convinced us that the cell body of the amebas is generally separated from target cells by an extracellular space 10–20 nm wide. Direct contact between these cell types seems to be established mainly through basal filopodia. These observations tend to support the notion that this particular type of pseudopodium is involved in attachment. The possibility that contact lysis is also mediated through filopodia has not been proved. This problem is difficult to solve since filopodia other than those associated with the uroid are below the resolution of the light microscope, and thus its pathogenic role cannot be directly established with the use of time-lapse microcinematography.

The majority of the largest filopodia, thick enough to be seen with the light microscope, are associated with the uroid (Figures 39 and 40), a fixed, refractile feature located in the posterior region of trophozoites engaged in active progression, to which foreign particles, cells, and bacteria attach. Time-lapse microcinematography clearly confirms that particles become firmly attached to the uroid region. Whether the uroid participates in endocytic (Lushbaugh and Pittman 1979) or exocytic (Hopkins and Warner 1946; Zaman 1961) processes remains to be determined. The uroid of motile trophozoites resembles the uropod of moving lymphocytes and neutrophils. The uropod appears in immunologically activated lymphocytes where it may be the site of interaction with target cells.

One of the surface specializations of *E. histolytica* trophozoites has raised considerable interest during recent years, in view of its possible role as the mechanism of parasite aggression. The so-called surface-active lysosomes were described by Eaton et al. (1969, 1970) as cup-shaped depressions, 0.1 to 2.0 μm in diameter, located beneath membrane-bound vacuoles. The surface cups were portrayed as frequently having a "frond-like outgrowth" protruding from the central region of the surface invagination. This was

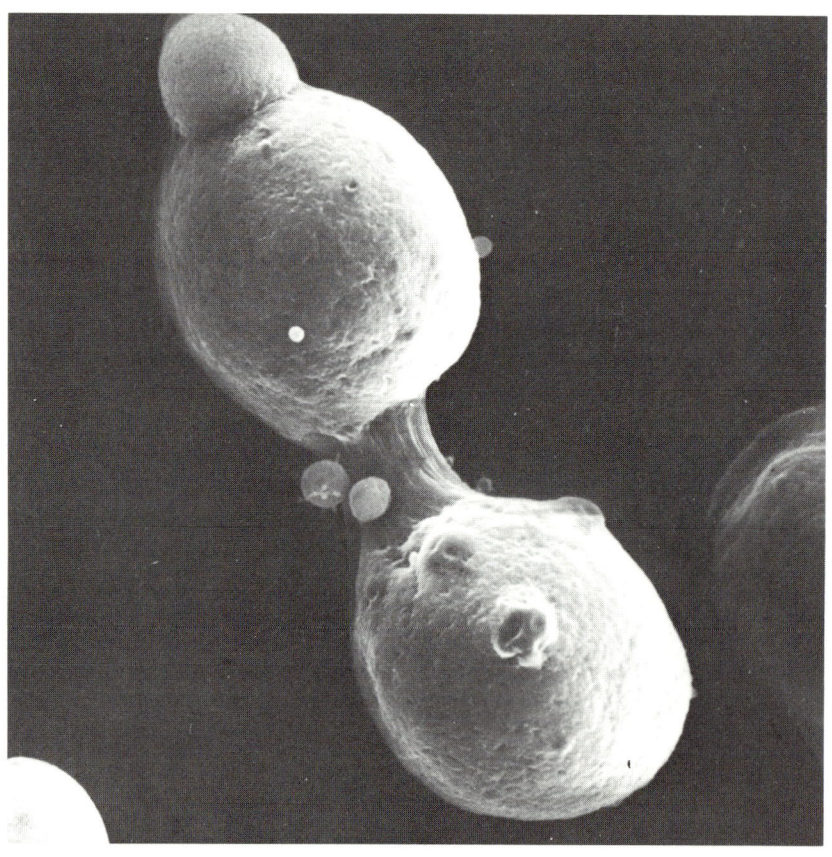

Figure 41. Scanning electron micrograph of a dividing trophozoite. During cell division, amebas show no filopodia. X 4,000.

supposed to act as a trigger after contact with a target cell, followed by the liberation of lytic enzymes and the ensuing lysis of the contacting cells. These entities were considered by various workers to represent the structural basis of the cytopathic activity of *E. histolytica,* and soon were reported in trophozoites obtained from cultures (Feria-Velasco and Treviño 1972; Proctor and Gregory 1973) and from colonic (Proctor and Gregory 1972) and liver (Treviño et al 1970) material. The presence of acid phosphatase at the limiting membrane of the surface vacuoles was reported by Eaton et al (1970). Lushbaugh et al (1976) verified that the enzyme activity is concentrated in the membrane of the vacuoles rather than being in soluble form in the lumen. Although the concept of contact lysis mediated by a specific "organelle" is attractive because of its simplicity, surface-active lysosomes have not been found in trophozoites of *E. histolytica* obtained from lesions (El-Hashimi and Pittman 1970; Griffin and Juniper 1971; Griffin 1972); in contrast, they have been found in nonpathogenic amebas such as *E. coli* and *E. moshkovskii* (Rondanelli et al. 1974). Serial sectioning has revealed that the trigger corresponds, in fact, to a filopodium (Deas and Miller 1977), and Lushbaugh and Pittman (1979) confirmed this observation using high voltage electron microscopy of thick sections. At present, there is no evidence to relate these filopodia and their associated vacuoles to contact lysis; as an alternative, they have been suggested as being involved in endocytosis (Rondanelli et al. 1977; Lushbaugh and Pittman 1979). In dividing amebas, filopodia are generally absent (Figure 41).

2.4 The Nucleus

The nucleus is generally inconspicuous when amebas are studied with bright field optics, but becomes clearly apparent when visualized with phase contrast or Nomarski interference optics. The latter is the method best suited for the light microscopic study of living trophozoites (Chévez et al. 1972a,b). In iron hematoxylin-stained preparations, the nucleus of the trophic form of *E. histolytica* is 4–7 μm in diameter (Figure 1). The nuclear membrane is outlined by a thin uniform layer of granules which gives the nucleus the appearance of a ring in optical section (Dobell 1919). Chromatin clumps are usually uniform in size and evenly distributed inside the nuclear membrane. However, in certain nuclei the chromatin may appear concentrated on one side as a crescentic mass. As shown by microcinematography, the nucleus has no fixed position in the cytoplasm, but moves freely and sometimes rotates rapidly. The karyosome or endosome is a small spherical mass, approximately 0.5 μm in diameter, located in the central part of the nucleus. In stained specimens, the endosome has a texture similar to that of peripheral chromatin, but it generally appears less dense (Figures 1 and 2). Between the endosome and the peripheral rim of chromatin, very little chromatin is found. The clear halo surrounding the karyosome and the "linin" network that gives the nucleus the well-known "cartwheel" appearance probably are fixation artifacts, since they are not found in amebas fixed in glutaraldehyde and osmium tetroxide and embedded in plastic resins, a method that gives much better preservation than the classical staining procedures. In many instances, the nuclei of *E. histolytica* trophozoites contain varying numbers of birefringent spheroidal bodies, 0.2 to 1.0 μm in diameter, evident with Nomarski or phase contrast light microscopic methods (Chévez et al. 1971).

Much confusion has been generated by giving names to nuclear structures visualized with hematoxylin. Singh (1952) points out that this is a matter of particular importance because the different genera and species among free-living and parasitic amebas have been defined largely on the basis of their nuclear structure and mode of nuclear division. This author has suggested that the term "peripheral chromatin" should be abolished, and the word "chromatin" applied only to those granules in the resting nucleus that stain with the Feulgen reaction and give rise to chromosomes during mitosis. This issue continues to be of concern since the fundamental basis of classification of *Entamoeba* remains its morphology, despite the structural simplicity of the organism (Neal 1966).

The nature of the nuclear components of *Entamoeba* during interphase has been explored using cytochemistry and radioautography to locate DNA- and RNA- containing regions; they appear to have a distribution different from the usual nuclear configuration of animal cells. The so-called "peripheral chromatin" gives a negative reaction to Feulgen staining; only the endosome and periendosomal particles are Feulgen-positive in *E. invadens* (Narasimhamurti 1964; Siddiqui and Rudzinska 1965). Pan and Geiman (1955) found that Feulgen-positive nuclear structures in *E. histolytica* appear during nuclear division, while in interphase, the nuclei usually remain negative. More recently, Albach et al.(1980) labeled *E. histolytica* with ^{3}H-thymidine and found the label randomly distributed in the nucleus, while RNA detected with a ^{3}H-uridine label accumulated mainly in the "peripheral chromatin." They suggest that "peripheral chromatin" is the counterpart of the eukaryotic nucleolus, while the endosome is a site of DNA condensation (heterochromatin).

The nuclear membrane is visualized with the electron microscope in freeze-fracture replicas (Figure 42) as a double membrane interrupted by numerous nuclear pores approximately 65 nm in diameter, with a mean density of 35 pores per square micrometer (Henley et al. 1976; Martínez-Palomo et al. 1976b; Injeyan et al. 1979). Both the pore density and distribution are irregular; only infrequently does an orderly arrangement of pores follow a hexagonal pattern. The fracture faces of the inner nuclear membrane show a rim surrounding the pore.

In thin sections studied with the transmission electron microscope, the "peripheral chromatin" may continuously line the nuclear envelope and is intensely electron-dense (Figure 43). At higher magnification the "chromatin" appears to be composed mainly of dense particles that resemble cytoplasmic ribosomes in diameter and density. The endosome appears as an irregular region of fibrogranular material, generally of lower electron-density than the "peripheral chromatin." "Button-like" intranuclear bodies are frequently found in sections of *Entamoeba* (Deutsch and Zaman 1959; Miller et al. 1961; Zaman 1973). More than thirty intranuclear bodies may be identified by light microscopy using differential interference optics (Chévez et al. 1971). The nature and function of the ubiquitous intranuclear bodies of *Entamoeba* are

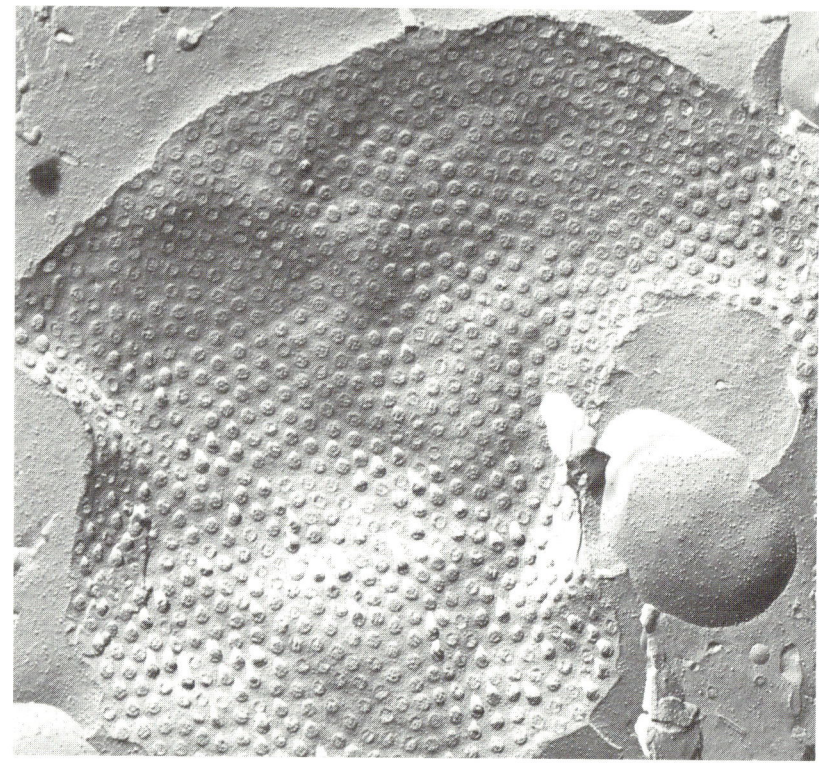

Figure 42. Nuclear membrane of a trophozoite in a freeze-fracture replica. X 25,000.

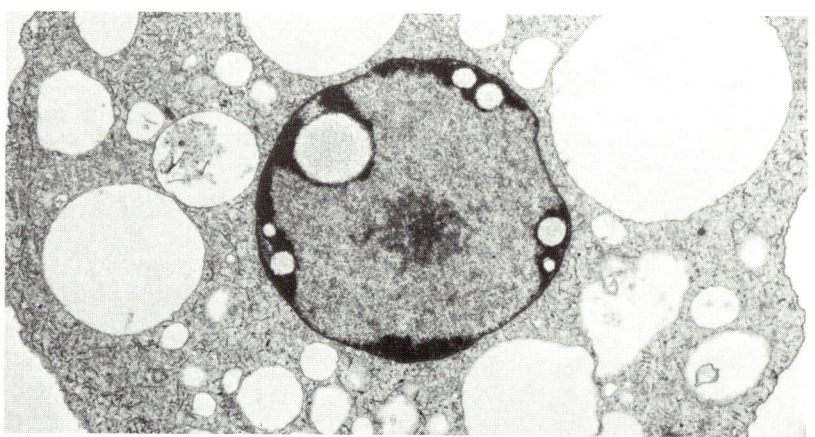

Figure 43. In a thin section of the nucleus of a trophozoite, the "peripheral chromatin," the karyosome, and various nuclear bodies are found. X 3,000.

not known. Only occasionally can they be found in the cytoplasm. They may be similar in function to the refractive granules described in *Tetrahymena pyriformis* that contain a large amount of lipid-like material as well as potassium, calcium, and magnesium phosphates, and appear to function as cellular buffers, maintaining constant levels of intracellular cations (Coleman et al 1973).

The mechanism of nuclear division of *E. histolytica* remains one of the least understood aspects of the biology of the parasite due to the small size of some of the nuclear components which approach the limits of resolution of the light microscope, and also because Heidenhain's iron hematoxylin technique, generally used by earlier workers, is unreliable since it involves destaining which cannot be standardized (Neal 1966). In spite of the efforts of various investigators (Mathis and Mercier 1961; Dobell 1919; Kofoid and Swezy 1925; Uribe 1926; Cleveland and Sanders 1930; Narasimhamurti 1964), the only fact that can be considered as settled is that nuclear division in *Entamoeba* proceeds without dissolution of the nuclear membrane. Most of the assertions of Dobell (1928) are still valid: "... I am still in doubt about the origin of the chromosomes and their exact number... I believe that the division is a mitosis of a peculiar kind, and that the chromosome number is probably constant: but what it really is I do not know... I am not confident about this and must therefore leave this important point in doubt."

We have recently obtained microcinematographic records of the nuclear division of cultured trophozoites of *E. invadens* and have corroborated that nuclear division proceeds without the dissolution of a nuclear envelope (Cervantes and Martínez-Palomo 1980). It is also evident that nuclear division takes place without the formation of distinct nuclear bodies which could be likened to typical eukaryotic chromosomes, thus confirming by microcinematography the observation of Dobell (1928) that no details of nuclear division can be made out in the living organism. Therefore, the entire mitotic process in *E. histolytica*, both in cysts and in trophozoites, remains to be settled. In 1-μm thick sections studied with light microscopy, fragmentation of the endosome into ill-defined small bodies has been found (Figure 44). The best way to clarify this subject would be to study thick sections of dividing cells with high voltage electron microscopy.

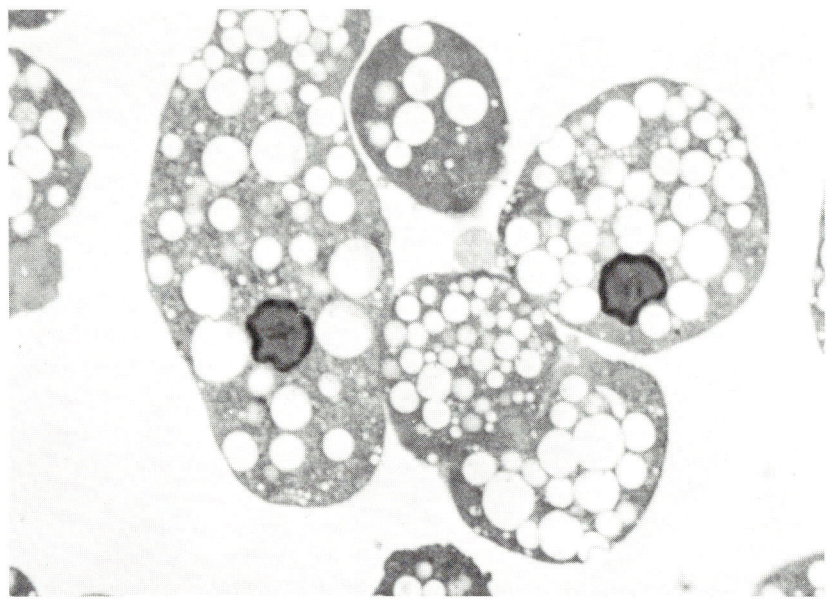

Figure 44. Light micrograph of trophozoites undergoing nuclear division. The endosome fragments fragment into small bodies. X 1,000.

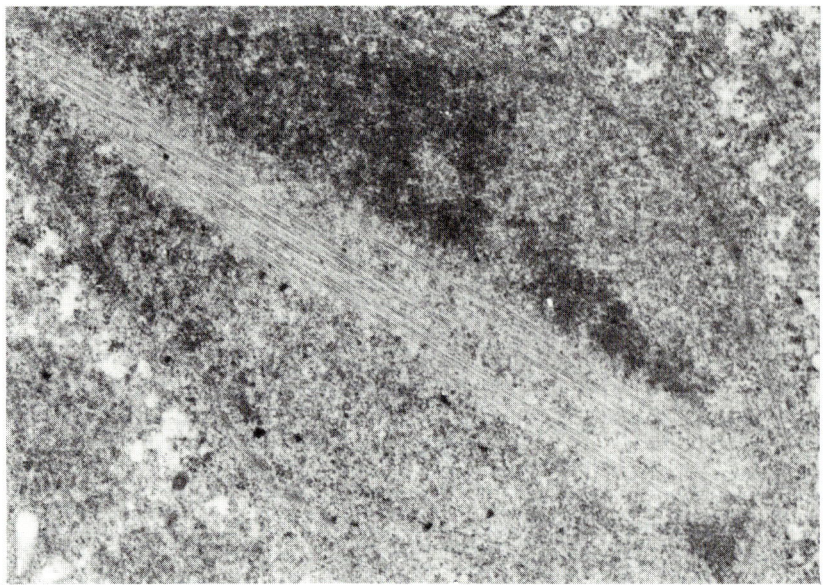

Figure 45. Nucleus of a trophozoite of *E. moshkovskii*. An intranuclear microtubular spindle is seen. X 35,000.

Very little information has been obtained on the nuclear division of *E. histolytica* using the standard techniques of transmission electron microscopy, since no centrioles, spindles, or chromosomes have been identified with certainty. Microtubular spindles have been reported in dividing *Entamoeba*. However, both reports (Gicquaud 1979; Injeyan et al. 1979) exclusively refer to amebas of the *E. histolytica*-Laredo type. Following a chance observation of microtubules in the dividing nuclei of *E. moshkovskii*, we have carried out a systematic search for microtubules in a variety of *Entamoeba* strains. They are easily demonstrated by electron microscopy in nuclei of *E. histolytica* strains isolated from human carriers, and from various strains of *Entamoeba* (*E. moshkovskii, E. histolytica*-Laredo type) that grow at room temperature (Figure 45). Microtubules are also present in the dividing nuclei of *E. histolytica* strains isolated from cases of invasive amebiasis, but for some reason microtubules are far more difficult to identify with certainty in these strains.

2.5 The Cyst

The life cycle of *E. histolytica* in the human host is unknown. Details on the complete life cycle of the parasite were obtained in a painstaking study carried out by Dobell (1928) in cultures of a strain of *E. histolytica* (K.28c) recovered from a monkey. Dobell stated that he had no proof that the ameba he called *E. histolytica* in *Macaca sinicus* was identical to the similar form in man "...but meantime I must ask the reader to accept this conclusion on insufficient evidence." In spite of this limitation, Dobell's observations remain the basis of our knowledge of the life cycle of *E. histolytica*, since essentially nothing has been added to his original description. The complete life cycle of *E. histolytica* consists of four consecutive stages; namely, the trophozoite, precyst, cyst, and metacystic ameba. The reader is referred to Dobell (1928) for details.

Trophozoites multiply by binary fission and encyst, producing typical quadrinucleate cysts after two successive nuclear divisions of uninucleate cysts. A single quadrinucleate metacystic ameba escapes from each cyst and produces eight uninucleate amebas after division. These observations were generally corroborated by Cleveland and Sanders (1930) in cultures, and by Tanabe (1934) in amebas isolated from human carriers and injected into white rats. Thus, Dobell's observations have been accepted and his diagrams are still reproduced in current monographs (Kudo 1966; Neal 1966).

The fact that encystation of cultured *E. histolytica* occurs only in xenic media has hampered the biochemical analysis of this process. Efforts to induce cyst formation in axenic medium have been only partially successful, and up to the present there is no method to induce encystation of *E. histolytica* as reliable as the one available for *E. invadens* (Rengpien and Bailey 1975). The latter system has provided a simple mean to analyze the differentiation of trophozoites into cysts, induced by a decrease in the osmolarity of the medium. It appears that a reduction in the medium tonicity is at least one of the environmental signals acting at the plasma membrane that trigger differentiation of *E. invadens* cysts (Bailey and Rengpien 1980). This system not only provides the opportunity to study the chemical changes taking place during cyst wall synthesis and deposition in *E. invadens*, but also is a remarkably simple and fast method for the exploration of the mechanisms of cellular differentiation in eukaryotes. An important contribution to the study of the biology of *E. histolytica* would be the discovery of a suitable medium to induce encystation of

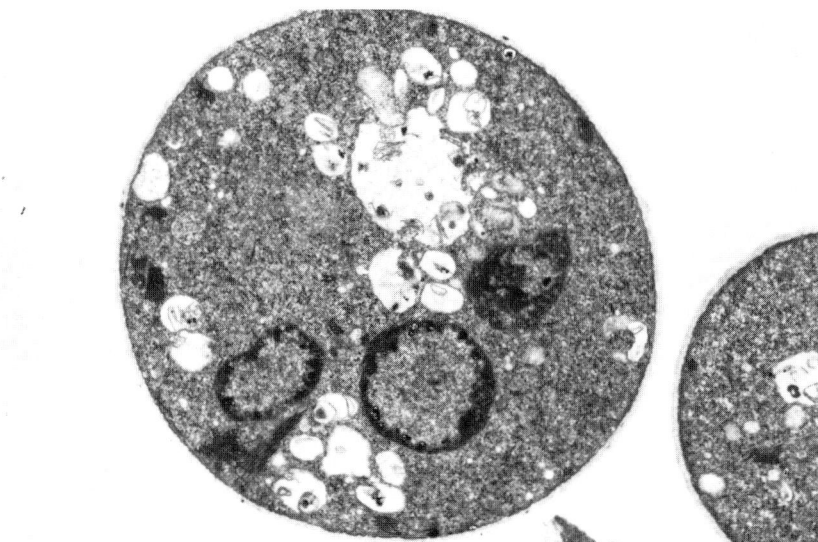

Figure 46. Low magnification of a thin section of a cyst. A cell wall covers the surface of the cyst. X 2,000.

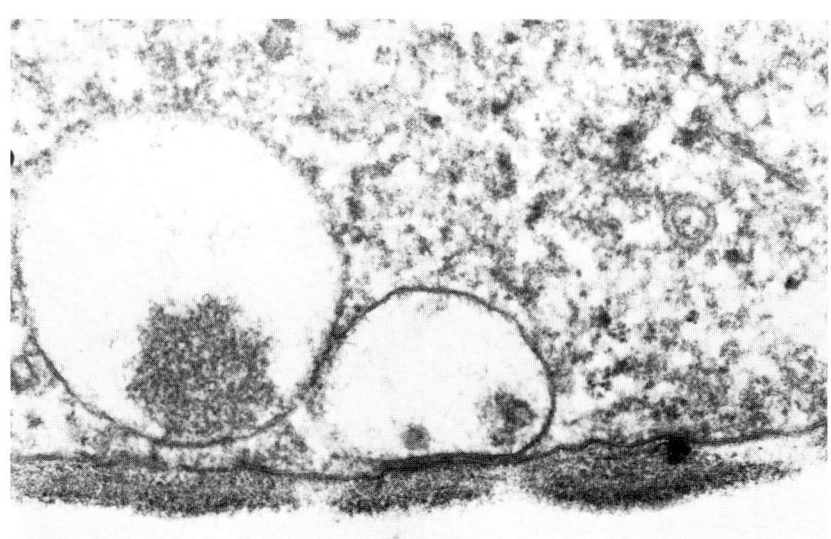

Figure 47. Vacuoles in close proximity to the plasma membrane of a cyst contain fibrillar material. X 64,000.

trophozoites, provided that the prolonged subculturing required for axenization would not result in an irreversible loss of the capacity of the amebas to differentiate into the resistant form.

Cysts are round or slightly oval in shape, ranging in diameter from 8 to 20 μm. In unstained smears they appear as hyaline bodies with a refractile wall. The cytoplasm is colorless and chromatoid bodies and nuclei are sometimes visible. One to four nuclei are clearly seen in specimens stained with iodine, which faintly stains chromatoid bodies as well. Glycogen stains reddish-brown. The "peripheral chromatin" lines the nuclear envelope and the karyosome may or may not have a central position. In general, the nuclei in interphase are similar to those of free forms. The size of the nucleus decreases as the number of nuclei is increased through division (Dobell 1919). With iron hematoxylin the cytoplasm appears vacuolated and glycogen deposits are visible as clear spaces, while chromatoid bodies are stained blue black and are rod-shaped with blunt or rounded ends (Spencer and Monroe 1961; McConnachie 1969).

When visualized with the electron microscope (Figure 46), the cyst wall which is 125–150 nm thick appears to be made of fibrillar elements 2–3 nm in diameter, giving rise to a tight mesh that may constitute several lamellae (Chávez et al 1978). The composition of the cyst wall has been studied in *E. invadens* by Arroyo-Begovich et al. (1980); it contains chitin as shown by chemical analysis and x-ray diffraction studies of purified preparations. The main sugars detected in acid hydrolysates from the walls are hexosamines.

The plasma membrane of *E. histolytica* cysts frequently shows deep invaginations. Polyribosomes and vacuoles containing dense fibrogranular material are closely apposed to the cytoplasmic face of the plasma membrane (Figure 47) (Chávez et al. 1978). The significance of this relationship in terms of the synthesis, transport, and deposition of cyst wall components remains to be determined. In thin sections, the cytoplasm and the nuclei of the cysts show a structural organization similar to that described above for trophozoites (Miller and Deas 1971; Proctor and Gregory 1973; Rondanelli et al. 1974). Glycogen deposits and polyribosomal crystals diminish as the cysts mature.

In spite of the fact that transmission of amebiasis depends on the formation of cysts, very few investigations have been carried out during the last decade on the encystation and excystation processes. *E. histolytica* cysts form in vivo when conditions are suitable for the formation of normal, relatively solid stools (McConnachie 1969). Some of the conditions that favor encystation in culture are the vigorous growth of the trophozoites before differentiation, "crowding," depletion of certain nutrients, and lowering of the tonicity of the medium. The finding of McConnachie (1969) that mass encystation occurs in the presence of diluted axenic growth medium revealed that bacteria or bacterial metabolites are not essential for the encystation of *E. invadens*; bacteria may act mainly to supply certain amino acids through the hydrolysis of proteins (Rengpien and Bailey 1975). Thus, one of the important results of the availability of axenic media for the culture of *Entamoeba* (Diamond 1968) has been the demonstration that bacteria are not essential for cyst formation. In addition, the use of axenic cultures has shown that the presence of bacteria in the culture is not essential for the expression of the pathogenicity of *E. histolytica* (Tanimoto et al 1971), as discussed in section 6.3.

CHAPTER 3
Biochemistry

3.1 Anaerobic and Aerobic Metabolism

The normal environment of the trophozoite form of *E. histolytica* is essentially anaerobic, and a low redox potential is required for its optimal growth in culture. *E. histolytica* has therefore been considered to be an obligate anaerobic parasite. However, amebas are able to consume oxygen, in spite of the lack of mitochondria (Wittner 1968; Montalvo et al 1971; Weinbach and Diamond 1974), and are able to grow in an atmosphere containing up to 5% oxygen. Below this concentration, amebas are able to detoxify the products of oxygen reduction (Band and Cirrito 1979).

The growth of *E. histolytica* requires specific carbohydrates; glucose or polymers that can be converted into glucose are essential (Charoenlarp et al 1968). Whether this specific requirement influences the in vivo invasive behavior of the parasite is unknown. In contrast to free-living amebas, the uptake of glucose by *E. histolytica* involves a specific transport system (Serrano and Reeves 1974) that accounts for approximately 100 times the amount of sugar incorporated by endocytosis. However, there may be important differences in the rate of endocytosis in different strains. In this respect, biochemical investigations of the parasite have referred to pinocytosis, taking into account the results of Serrano and Reeves (1974). These authors did not differentiate between the various forms of endocytosis; namely, phagocytosis, macropinocytosis, and micropinocytosis, all of which occur at varying rates in cultured trophozoites. The rate-limiting step of glucose consumption is the transport process itself and not its metabolism (Serrano and Reeves 1975).

The elucidation of the glycolytic pathway of *E. histolytica* has mainly been done in Reeve's laboratory. The catabolism of glucose by *E. histolytica* differs considerably from that of most eukaryotic animal cells in that unusual glycolytic enzyme systems operate, and mitochondria, cytochromes, and a citric acid cycle are not present. The products of glucose dissimilation vary according to whether metabolism occurs in the presence or absence of oxygen. The end products are CO_2, acetate, and ethanol; however, anaerobically, ethanol production surpasses that of acetate by a ratio of 3 to 1, whereas aerobically, the ratio is reversed. Hydrogen is produced only anaerobically. It has become apparent that amebic glycolysis has the same intermediates as the classic Embden-Meyerhof pathway, but that certain glycolytic enzymes are unusual; in addition, inorganic pyrophosphate, generally considered as an end product of metabolism, is used as an energy source although its free energy is less than that of ATP (reviewed by Weinbach et al 1976; Wood 1977). Under anaerobic conditions, glucose is almost quantitatively converted into ethanol and CO_2: 2 moles of glucose yield 4 moles of ethanol, 4 moles of CO_2, and 3 of ATP.

Glucose is phosphorylated by ATP to form glucose 6-phosphate through the action of a nonspecific hexokinase regulated by AMP. The conversion of fructose 6-phosphate to fructose 1,6-diphosphate is catalyzed by two phosphofructokinases. One of them, unique to *E. histolytica*, is specific for pyrophosphate rather than for ATP. Instead of pyruvate kinase which is absent in *E. histolytica*, a pyruvate phosphokinase specific for pyrophosphate converts phosphoenolpyruvate into pyruvate.

Pyruvate is first converted into acetylcoenzyme A and CO_2 in the conversion of pyruvate to ethanol. Acetylcoenzyme A synthetase produces ATP and acetate from acetyl-Co A and inorganic pyrophosphate, which represents a significant source of energy (Lo and Reeves 1978). Amebal ferredoxin may act as the primary electron acceptor in the anaerobic conversion of pyruvate, which would explain the production of hydrogen gas by amebas cultured with hydrogenase-containing bacteria, and the lack of hydrogen production in axenically grown cells (Tanowitz et al 1975). No organelle similar to the hydrogenosomes described in *Trichomonas* has been found in *Entamoeba*. The presence of the latter metabolic pathway would explain the sensitivity of the organism to 5-nitroimidazoles. Further details on the glycolytic pathway and intermediary metabolism can be found in Gutteridge and Coombs (1977). To summarize, the two striking elements that have been detected in the intermediary metabolism of *E. histolytica* are the unusually large concentration of intracellular inorganic pyrophosphate, and the presence of pyrophosphate-dependent kinases. This relatively primitive metabolic pattern may reflect an early divergence from the evolutionary pattern of development followed by other eukaryotic organisms (Gutteridge and Coombs 1977).

Glycogen, a conspicuous component of the cytoplasm of *E. histolytica* trophozoites, is their main energy source. Certain differences in the disposition of glycogen have been found between axenic and monoxenic amebas (Sharma et al 1970). The mechanism of glycogen synthesis in *E. histolytica* is not well understood since glycogen synthetase appears to be absent. Takeuchi et al (1977) have found that particulate glycogen present in axenic forms is joined by protein bridges. Glycogen synthesis may be mediated by a phosphorylase-saccharide membrane complex described by Takeuchi et al (1977). Most of the energy demands of *E. histolytica* are covered by glycolytic processes. However, as mentioned before, the parasite not only is able to utilize oxygen, but also has a very high affinity for it (Weinbach and Diamond 1974). The biological significance of respiration is unknown, but one possibility is that the oxidative enzymes of *E. histolytica* could act as a detoxification mechanism to remove oxygen from the parasite (Weinbach and Diamond 1974), which could be used by the ameba when faced with high oxygen concentrations during the invasive state.

Harlow et al (1976) have found a nicotinamide nucleotide transhydrogenase associated with a NADPH diaphorase that provides an anaerobic means of NADH oxidation, fundamentally different from the cytochrome-containing NADH oxidation system in mitochondria. They speculate that this enzyme could participate in energy conservation. The same group (Weinbach et al 1977) subsequently found diaphorase activity in *E. histolytica* that catalyzes the oxidation of NADPH, restoring NADP. Thus, transhydrogenase and diaphorase act in sequence to maintain the NADP required for glycolysis. The diaphorase-transhydrogenase system may account for a significant proportion of the respiration of the parasite, providing an anaerobic mechanism for regulating the redox state of nicotinamide nucleotides. The individual flavin species of *E. histolytica* have been studied by Lo and Reeves (1979). Flavin mononucleotide is the major flavin; flavin-adenine dinucleotide and riboflavin are present in lesser amounts.

As is obvious from the above mentioned observations, the metabolism of *E. histolytica* is puzzling. This protozoan is an anaerobe with peculiar glycolytic enzymes found in certain bacteria, that also has the capacity to avidly consume oxygen and to grow at low oxygen concentrations. This protean metabolism may be an advantage, enabling the parasite to shift from the environment of the intestinal lumen at low oxygen pressure to a completely different one encountered when it invades solid organs with an abundant blood supply. Whether the unusual characteristics of the amebal metabolism can be exploited for the rational design of safe and effective antiamebic drugs is still unknown.

3.2 Membrane Composition

The understanding of the complex phenomena occurring during host-parasite interactions in amebiasis requires knowledge of the chemical composition of the parasite membranes. For example, the characterization of the immunological reaction of the host in invasive amebiasis and of the membrane interactions involved in the cytopathic effect of *E. histolytica* on target cells have to take into account the composition of the plasma membrane and the internal membranes of the protozoan.

The exploration into the biochemistry of amebas began with free-living species such as *Acanthamoeba castellanii*. The membranes of this protozoan have an unusual composition: the number of polypeptides is low, and a sizeable amount of the membrane is made up a phospholipoglycan (Korn 1975), in contrast to the comparatively high number of proteins and the complex lipid composition of most eukaryotic membranes.

Only recently has the biochemistry of *Entamoeba* membranes been explored. Initially, studies have concentrated on *E. invadens*, a parasite of reptiles, because this *Entamoeba* species grows at room temperature under less stringent requirements than those necessary for the collection of large amounts of trophozoites of *E. histolytica*. An analysis of the total lipids of *E. histolytica* trophozoites showed that $60-70^0/0$ are composed of phospholipids, while cholesterol is a major component of the nonsaponifiable fraction (Sawyer et al 1967). Later, the fatty acid composition of *E. histolytica* was found to be similar to that of *E. invadens* (Cerbón and Flores 1981).

Lipids of *Entamoeba* species have been studied both in whole extracts of trophozoites (McLaughlin and Meerovitch 1975b; Cerbón and Flores 1981) and in isolated plasma membrane and internal membrane fractions (Aley et al 1980). In general, the lipid composition varies qualitatively and quantitatively from that of mammalian cells; in particular, ethanolamine-containing lipids predominate over those lipids containing choline. Extracts contain an unusual phospholipid ceramide aminoethyl phosphonate (CAEP) and phosphatidylcholine is also present in large amounts (McLaughlin and Meerovich 1975b; Cerbón and Flores 1981). Other phospholipids include phosphatidic acid, phosphatidylinositol, phosphatidylserine, and sphingomyelin. The phospholipid composition of the plasma membrane differs from that of intact cells and internal vesicles in that phosphatidylcholine levels are lower in the plasma membrane and CAEP is increased (Aley et al 1980).

The unusual composition of the membrane lipids of *Entamoeba* in general, and *E. histolytica* in particular, could be related to the requirement for both remarkable plasticity and stability (Cerbón and Flores 1981). In addition, the presence of ceramide aminoethylphosphonate may confer important biological advantages since this compound is resistant to hydrolysis, and amebas are able to efficiently resynthesize ceramide ethanolaminephosphate. Amebas may therefore be more resistant to hydrolytic enzymes in the digestive tract and may also resist amebic phospholipase action, which has been suggested as one of the possible means of aggression by the parasite (McCaul and Bird 1977).

Analysis of the protein composition of *E. histolytica* membranes is difficult because the marker enzymes used to differentiate plasma membrane from internal membrane fractions may not be present, and because their potent proteolytic activity tends to degrade polypeptides during the isolation procedure.

McLaughlin and Meerovitch (1975a,b) identified at least nine distinct polypeptides in a fraction enriched with plasma membranes, and found a potent membrane-bound acid phosphohydrolase. In a membrane fraction isolated from amebal homogenates, assumed to correspond to the plasma membrane and digestive vacuoles of *E. histolytica*, Serrano et al.(1977) found acid phosphatase activity associated with the membranes. Sialic acid was absent in all fractions of *E. invadens* (McLaughlin and Meerovitch 1975b). Serrano et al.(1977) were unable to detect glycoprotein bands by periodic acid-Schiff staining of gels, and found eight prominent peaks in polyacrylamide gel electrophoresis of isolated *E. histolytica* fractions. Later, Aley et al.(1980) obtained purified fractions of *E. histolytica* plasma membranes using concanavalin A as a stabilizing agent. In those fractions, they detected at least twelve proteins ranging between 12,000–200,000 MW. Several of the polypeptides were judged to be glycoproteins because of their ability to bind to columns of insolubilized concanavalin A and to be eluted by mannose.

The presence of carbohydrate-containing components in the plasma membrane of *E. histolytica* was detected by ultrastructural cytochemistry (Pinto da Silva et al. 1975). Mannose or glucose residues on the cell surface were identified by the agglutination of pathogenic strains of *E. histolytica* with concanavalin A, and inhibition of the reaction with alpha-methyl mannoside (Martínez-Palomo et al. 1973). Concanavalin A receptors were detected at the ultrastructural level with the use of the sequential concanavalin A-peroxidase-benzidine reaction (Trissl et al. 1977) or iodine-labeled concanavalin A (Calderón and Martínez-Palomo, unpublished observations).

The method employed by Aley et al. (1980) to isolate plasma membrane-enriched preparations permits both the study of the antigenic components of the cell surface, and the possible chemical and antigenic differences between pathogenic and nonpathogenic strains of *E. histolytica*. A better characterization of the most significant membrane antigens will be achieved in the near future with the use of monoclonal antibodies.

3.3 Growth and Differentiation

Most of the recent efforts devoted to understanding the processes of growth and differentiation of *E. histolytica* have focused on the development of better media for the cultivation of the parasite. Cultivation of fecal material for the isolation and growth of *E. histolytica* is of special diagnostic value, enabling the confirmation of a positive but doubtful microscopic diagnosis, or the isolation of the organism when other techniques have failed. Several methods are available that give excellent results in the hands of the experienced worker (Robinson 1968; Edelman and Springarn 1977).

For research purposes, the long-sought target was the development of axenic cultures, finally obtained through Diamond's perseverance (1961, 1968). The availability of axenic cultures has had a significant impact on the realization of biochemical and immunological investigations of *E. histolytica*. Here it will suffice to mention that both the TP-S-1 monophasic medium (trypticase-panmede-serum; Diamond 1968) and the new TYI-S-33 medium (trypticase-yeast extract-iron-serum; Diamond et al 1978a) give excellent results. Since both media are extremely complex in composition, further improvements should be in the direction of developing a better-defined medium, and ultimately, in the design of a chemically defined medium capable of supporting the growth and differentiation of *E. histolytica*.

Entamoeba histolytica can be cultured only in highly complex undefined liquid media (Diamond 1968; Diamond et al 1978a; Diamond 1980). Amebas can also be grown as colonies from single cells in semisolid agar suspension (Gillin and Diamond 1978). The latter method is particularly useful for quantifying cell viability. Recent efforts to obtain a defined culture medium have demonstrated that cysteine, ascorbic acid, albumin, and various vitamins are required (Gillin and Diamond 1980). In a medium containing these components plus various salts and Tris-HCl buffer, amebas may remain motile for 12 to 24 hours. It has been found that amebas deprived of cysteine remain rounded, fail to attach, and soon lyse; the absence of ascorbic acid also reduces the ability of the amebas to attach to glass surfaces. The requirement for cysteine in the presence of ascorbic acid is highly specific. These components not only protect the amebas from oxygen, but also are indispensable when the cells are placed in a nitrogen atmosphere (Gillin and Diamond 1980). Growth of *E. histolytica* requires riboflavin, for which a high-affinity transport system exists (Lo and

Reeves 1979). Furthermore, several precursors of nucleic acids have been shown to stimulate the growth of amebas (Reeves and West 1980), and transport systems for adenine and adenosine have been found in *E. histolytica* (Boonlayangoor et al 1978). As mentioned previously, the growth of *E. histolytica* also requires glucose or polymers that can be converted into glucose; the rate-limiting step of glucose consumption is the transport process (Serrano and Reeves 1975).

Anyone who has had some experience with the axenic cultivation of *E. histolytica* will agree that the organism is certainly fastidious in its growth under in vitro conditions, being sensitive to changes in batches of serum and other components of the media. An additional problem much too often overlooked is the susceptibility of *E. histolytica* trophozoites to changes in temperature, centrifugation, repeated washes in balanced solutions, etc., that has induced several investigators to concentrate on the more resistant *E. invadens*, only to be faced later with the problem of extrapolating the results to *E. histolytica*.

Diamond's new medium (1978a) gives greater yields and more uniform growth with smaller inocula than his previous axenic medium. A 100-fold increase in the number of amebas is obtained after approximately 72 hours of incubation. In general, reculturing is carried out every 72 hours with *E. histolytica*, and each week with room temperature strains. The required low oxygen concentration, which is less than that present in air, is obtained by using screw vials filled almost completely with media. Plastic culture bottles may be toxic because of the oxygen dissolved in the plastic walls (Band and Cirrito 1979), although in our experience this problem is encountered only exceptionally. High concentrations of oxygen will kill the cells, but they become insensitive to the action of oxygen at low temperature (Gillin and Diamond 1980). The optimal temperature for the growth of *E. histolytica* is between 35.5 and 37.0 °C (Gillin and Diamond 1980).

Recent refinements include the use of semisolid media for cloning (Gillin and Diamond 1978), and the development of a maintenance medium free of serum and unidentified components (Gillin and Diamond 1980) that maintains viable amebas for several hours.

Several investigators have cast doubt on the validity of using axenic cultures of *E. histolytica* in experimental amebiasis, since it was generally believed that amebas lost their virulence under axenic conditions. However, it has been clearly demonstrated that axenic amebas are able to induce sterile liver abscesses in hamsters (Tanimoto et al 1971) and ulceration of the intestinal mucosa of the guinea pig cecum (Diamond et al 1978b). Furthermore, the degree of virulence of different strains of pathogenic *E. histolytica* is correlated with the degree of their cytopathic effect on epithelial cultures (Martínez-Palomo et al 1980b).

An important question is whether all *E. histolytica* strains can be grown in axenic media. Although nonpathogenic strains of the Laredo type and *E. moshkovskii* grow very well in axenic cultures, no reports have appeared on the successful axenic cultivation of strains of *E. histolytica* isolated from asymptomatic carriers. The strains isolated by Bos (1975) may not be carrier strains, since the carrier state was not clearly ascertained. Recently, De la Torre, Tanimoto, and Martínez-Palomo (unpublished observations) have isolated two strains from well-characterized asymptomatic carriers (strains HM29:IMSS and HM35:IMSS). Both strains, grown in axenic medium, have been shown to be avirulent since they do not produce liver abscesses in newborn hamsters after direct inoculation of up to 50,000 amebas. Further studies are needed to define the different culture requirements of pathogenic and nonpathogenic amebas.

The differentiation of *E. histolytica* into cysts, including encystation, multiplication, and excystation, remains one of the least understood aspects of the biology of the parasite. Considering that the cyst is the resistant form that enables *E. histolytica* to survive the adverse conditions outside of the intestinal tract, and is therefore responsible for the transmission of the infection, it is surprising how little attention has been paid to this particular issue. A partial explanation for the apparent lack of interest in the differentiation of *E. histolytica* is the inability up to now to induce cyst formation in axenic cultures. For this reason, most of the few but interesting new results related to this topic have been obtained with the use of cultures of *E. invadens* that will easily encyst under axenic conditions (McConnachie 1969; Rengpien and Bailey 1975).

The differentiation of the trophic form of *E. histolytica* into the cyst form appears to be triggered by environmental factors. Initially, encystation of cultured *E. invadens* appeared to be related to local depletion of carbohydrate sources and to changes in the osmolarity of the medium (Balamuth 1962). Cyst formation is accompanied by a slowing down of movement, cessation of endocytosis, the gradual appearance of glycogen, and the progressive fragmentation of chromatoid bodies. Encystation occurs in vivo when conditions are suitable for the formation of normal, relatively solid stools; no cysts are found in acute dysenteric forms of amebiasis.

At first, Thepsuparungskikul et al (1971) considered bacterial metabolites or the action of bacteria upon serum components to be essential for the encystation of *E. invadens*. These authors found no clear-cut correlation between cell division or crowding and encystation. However, in support of the observations of McConnachie (1969), they demonstrated that mass encystation occurs in hypotonic axenic medium, thus ruling out the alleged essential role of bacteria in encystation as well as the theory that it is a response to nutrient depletion. The applicability of these observations in regard to cyst formation in the human intestinal tract is not known. Krishna Murti (1975) has found that encystation of *Hartmannella culberstoni* is initiated by biogenic amines that bind to the plasma membrane and activate adenylate cyclase, inducing the activity of cellulose synthetase and the formation of a cellulose cyst wall. Under similar conditions, *E. histolytica* failed to encyst and did not bind biogenic amines.

The process of excystation has been the subject of detailed observations. The reader is referred to the fascinating description of the excystation of *E. histolytica* made by Dobell (1928).

Until recently, practically nothing was known concerning the chemical composition of the cell wall of *E. histolytica* cysts. Based on cytochemical evidence, McConnachie (1969) suggested that it contained a carbohydrate-protein complex. Arroyo-Begovich et al (1980) have found by direct chemical analysis and x-ray diffraction that chitin constitutes the microfibrillar component of the cyst wall of *E. invadens*.

Further work is needed to determine the biosynthetic pathways and cellular components involved in the process of cyst wall formation. The differentiation of the cyst, prompted by a change in the osmolarity of the medium, represents a fascinating system in which to probe the nature of the biochemical events leading from a change in the surface membrane to the expression of a specific phenotypic differentiation. In addition, elucidation of the mechanism of the biosynthesis of the cell wall and information on the unexplored process of excystation could possibly suggest biological means by which the cell cycle of *E. histolytica* could be interrupted. For example, the specific inhibition of the synthesis of the wall by chemical agents could interfere with the enzyme reactions necessary for cyst development, but not affect the metabolism of the host.

CHAPTER 4
Species of *Entamoeba*

The genus *Entamoeba* comprises several species of human parasites: *E. histolytica* Schaudinn, 1903; *E. hartmanni* von Provazek, 1912; *E. coli* (Grassi 1879) Hickson, 1909; and *E. gingivalis* (Gros 1849) Smith and Barrett, 1914. Of these amebas, *E. histolytica* is the only important cause of disease. The classification of the species of *Entamoeba* is based on the number of nuclei in their mature cysts, either eight, four, or one (Neal 1966). *E. coli* belongs to the octonucleate cyst group. Uninucleate cysts of *E. polecki*, a common parasite in pigs, have occasionally been found in man. In the quadrinucleate cyst group, *E. histolytica* can be differentiated from *E. hartmanni* on the basis of the diameter of the cysts, which are less than 10 μm in the latter. In addition to this genetically determined difference in cyst size, *E. hartmanni* has some distinct morphological features and is not pathogenic. Therefore, this ameba has received the status of a species separate from *E. histolytica* (Burrows 1957; Freedman and Elsdon-Dew 1959; Neal 1966; W.H.O. 1969). With the recognition of *E. hartmanni* as a species, the term "small race" should no longer be employed to designate it. A fourth group is formed by a single species, *E. gingivalis*, for which no cyst form is known.

"Typical" *E. histolytica* include both the minuta or cyst-forming phase and the large invasive erythrophagocytic amebas found in invasive amebiasis. The minuta form is considered to be the essential stage of *E. histolytica* since it is the only one capable of forming cysts, whereas the large hematophagous ameba has no place in the normal life cycle... "by exceeding the bounds of hospitality (they fail to) show any regard for its host nor for its own sustained posterity. Unchecked, such invasion may lead to death of the host and racial suicide for themselves" (Elsdon-Dew 1979).

Another type of quadrinucleate *Entamoeba* are the *E. histolytica*-like Laredo-type amebas; despite their nonpathogenicity, ability to grow at room temperature and to survive hypotonicity, and their distinct isoenzyme pattern, they have not yet been classified as a separate species. Therefore, using simple criteria such as size and growth at low temperatures, *E. hartmanni* and Laredo amebas can be distinguished. In addition, *E. moshkovskii*, present in sewage in various areas of the world, shows many properties in common with the Laredo organisms, except that it is a free-living ameba. A summary of the main features of various quadrinucleated *Entamoeba* species is presented in Table 1.

Since *E. histolytica* and *E. hartmanni* are usually distinguished by measuring the diameter of the cysts of the trophic forms, *E. hartmanni* still goes unreported in many clinical laboratories that do not routinely measure intestinal amebas. Similarly, Laredo strains pass unnoticed unless isolated amebas are cultured and the ability of the isolate to grow at low temperatures is tested.

During the first half of this century, one of the most heated topics in human protozoology was whether different species of "*E. histolytica*" exist. Variations in size, virulence, and growth temperature were reported in different strains. Hoare (1952) and Elsdon-Dew (1968, 1971) have given highly readable historical accounts of this debate.

Two of the most puzzling aspects of the biology of *E. histolytica* are the unexplained variability in its pathogenic potential and the restriction of human invasive amebiasis to certain geographical areas in spite of the worldwide distribution of the parasite. When the colonic environment is suitable, the parasite survives and usually remains in the lumen as a commensal, multiplying and forming cysts without producing obvious pathological effects. However, in certain areas of the world such as Mexico, Western and Southeastern Asia, and Southern Africa (Elsdon-Dew 1971), infection with *E. histolytica* is more commonly associated with the invasive form of the disease, manifested as amebic dysentery or liver abscesses.

TABLE 1

DIFFERENCES BETWEEN SOME QUADRINUCLEATED ENTAMOEBA SPECIES

	E. histolytica	E. invadens	E. hartmanni	E. h. Laredo	E. moshkovskii
ORIGIN	human	reptiles	human	human	sewage
PATHOGENICITY	(——— pathogenic ———)	(——— pathogenic ———)	(——— nonpathogenic ———————————)		
GROWTH:					
Temperature[1,2]	37°C	27°C	37°C	(——— 27°C ———)	
Max. dilution[1,3]	0	1:16	1:4	1:64	1:64
Agar[4]	(——— high CFE ———)			(——— low CFE ———)	
EMETINE[5,6]	sensitive			(——— less sensitive ———————————)	
ISOENZYMES[7,8]	specific	(——— different from E. h. ———)			
ANTIGENS[3,9]	specific	(——— different from E. h. ———)			
PROTEINS[10]	specific			(——— specific ———)	
DNA[11,12]	specific	(——— different from E. h. ———————————————————————)			

E. h. = E. histolytica; CFE = Cloning forming efficiency.

[1]Richards et al. 1966; [2]Neal 1966; [3]Goldman 1969; [4]Gillin and Diamond 1978; [5]Albach et al. 1966; [6]Entner et al. 1962; [7]Reeves and Bischoff 1968; [8]Sargeaunt et al. 1980; [9]Krupp 1966; [10]Saíd and López-Revilla 1978; [11]Gelderman et al. 1971; [12]López-Revilla and Gómez 1978.

4.1 Strain Variations

For more than five decades, experts on amebiasis have tried to explain the peculiar behavior of *E. histolytica* on the basis of three different hypotheses:

a) *E. histolytica* is a single species that always produces intestinal ulcerations which may or may not give rise to clinical manifestations.

b) *E. histolytica* comprises two different species of morphologically similar amebas; one is pathogenic (*E. dysenteriae*) and the other is not (*E. dispar*).

c) The species *E. histolytica* is composed of an unknown number of different strains. They may act as commensals in the intestinal lumen (carrier state or lumenal amebiasis), or may behave as pathogenic forms that produce ulceration of the large intestine and give rise to symptoms (invasive amebiasis).

4.1.1 The unicist hypothesis

Dobell (1919), who stated that "*E. histolytica* is always a destroyer of tissue, but by no means always a producer of disease," thought that there is normally there is a state of equilibrium between the host and the parasite; the latter feeds at the expense of the host's tissues, but these regenerate and do not give rise to symptoms ("every healthy carrier has the lining of his large bowel more or less ulcerated"; Dobell 1919). Later, he modified his view and suggested that *E. histolytica* could be a commensal (Dobell 1931). D'Antoni (1952) and Faust et al. (1970) have strongly favored the earlier hypothesis. According to Faust et al (1970), no strain of *E. histolytica* has been found to be nonpathogenic in susceptible experimental animals; invasive amebiasis arises when amebas with a low pathogenic index, that normally erode the mucosal surface, multiply in a host that develops a low threshold of resistance, or else when a human host is infected with strains of a higher pathogenic index. This hypothesis, called "promethean" by Elsdon-Dew (1968), one of his most energetic and best-informed opponents, can now be dismissed since it fails to explain the existence of important geographic differences in the incidence of invasive amebiasis, and because true asymptomatic carriers show no evidence of intestinal invasion, as demonstrated by rectosigmoidoscopy and negative serology.

4.1.2 The dualistic hypothesis

Brumpt (1949) offered a very different explanation for the apparent erratic behavior of *E. histolytica*. On epidemiological grounds, he proposed that the high incidence of invasive forms of amebiasis in some geographical locations is due to the prevalence of a pathogenic species of *Entamoeba* in those regions, which he called *E. dysenteriae*, following the designation of Councilman and Lafleur (1891). In areas where amebic infection is restricted to lumenal amebiasis without symptoms attributable to invasion, the prevalent parasite would belong to a nonpathogenic species, *E. dispar* (Brumpt 1925). Both species were considered by Brumpt to be morphologically similar, differing mainly in their pathogenicity to man. *E. dispar* would have a cosmopolitan distribution, whereas *E. dysenteriae* would be restricted to warm climates (Brumpt 1949). Brumpt (1949) reviewed the available data on the incidence of *E. histolytica* infections in various countries and concluded that if all isolates of *E. histolytica* belonged to the same species, the same ameba would be pathogenic in one in every five individuals in the Philippines and in one in every two million in England.

Brumpt's dualistic hypothesis concerning the nature of pathogenic and nonpathogenic forms of *E. histolytica* in man found support only among French parasitologists; Anglo-Saxon investigators initially paid little if any attention to his views. Neal (1966) reviewed Brumpt's evidence and concluded that since, according to his experience, the virulence of *E. histolytica* is an unstable characteristic, it would be unwise to give specific status to this factor. Hoare (1952) suggested that *E. dispar* is merely the minuta stage of *E. histolytica* appearing in symptomless carriers. Recently, however, there has been renewed interest in the possible existence of pathogenic and nonpathogenic species of *E. histolytica* (Elsdon-Dew 1979; Sargeaunt and Williams 1979; Sargeaunt et al 1980b). This issue is of considerable importance, not only as an explanation of the intriguing geographical differences in the distribution of invasive amebiasis, but also because, if true, treatment could be limited to only those patients harboring pathogenic amebas (Anonymous 1979).

The results of Sargeaunt's recent studies (Sargeaunt and Williams 1978, 1979, Sargeaunt et al. 1978, 1980a,b) described in section 4.4, indicate that the isoenzyme patterns of *E. histolytica* isolated from cases of human dysentery differ from those of isolates obtained from asymptomatic carriers, thus raising the possibility that different genetic types of amebas may be responsible for invasive and lumenal amebiasis.

4.1.3 The pluralistic hypothesis

The hypothesis prevalent in the literature during the last two decades holds that *E. histolytica* comprises an unknown number of different strains with varying degrees of virulence. The most virulent ones are restricted to regions where invasive amebiasis is prevalent, while those of low virulence have a worldwide distribution. Some strains act as commensals living in the intestinal lumen without producing ulceration; others behave as virulent forms, the virulence of which varies according to the specific strain (Kuenen and Swellengrebel 1913; Hoare 1952; Van Steenis 1957; Swellengrebel 1961; Van Thiel 1961; Neal 1966; Elsdon-Dew 1968; W.H.O. 1969). Crowding and repeated fecal transmission would promote rapid reinfection that would in turn increase the virulence of *E. histolytica* (Swellengrebel 1961). *E. histolytica* would then be only one species embracing a spectrum of strains of varying virulence.

4.2 *Entamoeba histolytica*-like Amebas

Since 1956, an increasing number of *E. histolytica*-like, Laredo-type amebas have been isolated, most of them from presumptive asymptomatic carriers. These isolates morphologically similar to typical *E. histolytica*, differ mainly in their capacity to multiply at room temperature and to withstand hypotonic solutions (Richards et al. 1966; Goldman 1969). They are further characterized by their very low pathogenicity to man and laboratory animals (Rosas and Najarian 1965), increased resistance to emetine and various antibiotics (de Carneri 1959; Entner and Most 1962), and minor antigenic differences from *E. histolytica*. Reeves and Bischoff (1968) and Sargeaunt et al. (1980a) have strengthened the notion that *E. histolytica*-like, Laredo-type amebas belong to a species different from the classical *E. histolytica* strains by demonstrating that the former have electrophoretic isoenzyme patterns distinct from the latter. In addition, the Laredo amebas have been found to possess physiological properties very similar to *E. moshkovskii*, except that the latter is free-living and the former is parasitic (Goldman 1969; Sargeaunt et al. 1980a). This resemblance tends to confirm the suggestion of Goldman (1969) that *E. moshkovskii* is actually an ameba of the Laredo type, only incidentally encountered in free-living environments because of its wide temperature and osmolarity tolerances. It appears then that Laredo-type *E. histolytica* and *E. moshkovskii* belong to a species different from *E. histolytica*. As proposed by Goldman (1969), there is some possibility that Brumpt's *E. dispar* may be the Laredo-type *E. histolytica*: "...we should be impressed by the fact that this (*E. dispar*) is an accurate, if incomplete, description of the Laredo-type strains now known" (Goldman 1969).

4.3 Differences Between Carrier and Invasive Strains

Under conditions in which carriers are strictly selected on the basis of negative clinical history, absence of macroscopic lesions demonstrated by rectosigmoidoscopy, and negative serology, carrier isolates of *E. histolytica* (strains HM7:IMSS, HM9:IMSS, HM29:IMSS, HM35:IMSS) grown in monoxenic or axenic cultures have been shown to be nonpathogenic when inoculated into the livers of adult or newborn hamsters (Tanimoto-Weki et al 1974; Martínez-Palomo, Tanimoto, and de la Torre, unpublished observations). Furthermore, carrier strains differ from invasive amebas in certain surface properties such as the tendency to agglutinate in the presence of concanavalin A (Martínez-Palomo et al. 1973). In our hands, pathogenicity is a relatively stable factor in axenic or monoxenic cultures of *E. histolytica*; the degree of virulence may slightly increase or decrease during prolonged subcultivation, but pathogenic strains remain capable of inducing liver abscesses following inoculation in the liver of hamsters, while those isolated from carriers consistently fail to induce hepatic lesions under the same conditions. These observations tend to support the notion that isolates of *E. histolytica* obtained from cases of invasive amebiasis are biologically different from carrier strains. In turn, the latter resemble the Laredo-type amebas. However, it cannot be concluded that carrier strains and Laredo strains belong to a single species comparable to *E. dispar* described by Brumpt (1925) because many carrier strains are not able to grow at room temperature.

Although carrier strains are different from invasive strains, there is still insufficient evidence to give them separate status as a species. The isolation of large numbers of strains from adequately defined carriers in various geographical regions, followed by the study of their pathogenicity, growth conditions, and isoenzyme patterns, will probably settle the issue of whether invasive and carrier strains of *E. histolytica* constitute two different species.

4.4 Biochemical Taxonomy

Two main biochemical approaches have been used to study the similarities and differences between various isolates of the *Entamoeba* group. Genotypic differences are determined by analyzing the DNA of *Entamoeba* cultures. Parameters such as total DNA per cell, base composition, and nucleotide sequences are studied because they are relatively fixed characteristics of individual species and have been successfully applied in the phylogenetic and taxonomic study of bacteria. In contrast, the study of isoenzymes involves the search for subtle molecular differences between various enzymes present in diverse cells, based on the charge, configuration, and molecular weight of the enzyme analyzed. This method cannot be used for diagnostic purposes because it is technically complex and because genotypic and phenotypic variations are found even within members of the typical *E. histolytica* group. However, the study of isoenzymes has demonstrated that the *Entamoeba* group is composed of biologically distinct species of amebas.

The DNA of typical *E. histolytica* is qualitatively and quantitatively different from that of *E. moshkovskii* and *E. histolytica*-like Laredo-type amebas (Gelderman et al 1971). Laredo types have the smallest amount of DNA per cell; *E. histolytica* has 5 times more; and *E. moshkovskii*, 10 times more. *E. histolytica* has the most repeated sequences, followed by *E. moshkovskii*; Laredo amebas have very few. The smaller genome size and the lack of repeated sequences has been taken as an indication that phylogenetically, *E. histolytica*-like, Laredo-type amebas are more primitive than the other two. Gelderman et al (1971) also analyzed the base composition of DNA from various members of the *Entamoeba* group. They characterized two typical genotypic species of *E. histolytica*. The base composition of *E. histolytica* was found to be different from that of *E. moshkovskii,* which is more closely related to *E. histolytica*-like amebas. *E. invadens* also has a different pattern. With the use of the buoyant density method, Reeves et al (1971) were able to find small but significant differences in the DNA of classical *E. histolytica* and *E. histolytica*-like strains. More recently, López-Revilla and Gómez (1978) have demonstrated fluctuations in the DNA content of various cultured strains of *Entamoeba* over a several month period. In spite of these variations, the DNA content of *E. histolytica* strains can be distinguished from that of *E. invadens* and *E. moshkovskii*.

The classification of *Entamoeba* species on the basis of the electrophoretic properties of their enzymes was pioneered by Reeves and Bischoff (1968) using cellulose acetate electrophoresis. The technique is based on the fact that amebic isomerases can be easily distinguished from bacterial enzymes; the method can therefore be used with xenic cultures, which means that the phenotypic features of cultures of *E. histolytica* recently isolated from feces can be determined. Reeves and Bischoff (1968) were able to demonstrate clear-cut differences between typical strains of *E. histolytica* and other entamoebas by studying five amebal enzymes in twenty-one different cultures. They determined the electrophoretic behavior of glucokinase, glucose phosphatase isomerase, phosphoglucomutase, malate dehydrogenase, and one NADP diaphorase.

The method was enthusiastically applied by Sargeaunt and Williams (1978, 1979; Sargeaunt et al. 1978, 1980a,b) in an effort to determine the phenotypic differences between pathogenic and nonpathogenic amebas. These authors studied three of the five enzymes employed by Reeves and Bischoff (1968). *E. coli* is enzymically completely different from typical *E. histolytica* (Sargeaunt and Williams 1978). In an initial survey of 85 cultures of *E. histolytica*, four groups were found based on their isoenzyme patterns. The exciting finding was that all eighteen stocks derived from patients with clinical amebiasis were found to be clustered in a single enzymic group (Sargeaunt and Williams 1979). This result suggested that invasive amebiasis is due to a biologically distinct species. Comparison of the enzyme patterns of *E. histolytica, E. hartmanni, Endolimax, Iodamoeba,* and *Dientamoeba* revealed that each species can be easily distinguished (Sargeaunt et al. 1980a). The finding of distinctive isoenzyme patterns in all of the above mentioned species of amebas which occur in the intestine of man was also relevant to the application of the technique in large-scale epidemiological studies. The occurrence of distinct patterns for *E. hartmanni* was particularly significant since it strengthened the current belief that this ameba is a species separate from *E. histolytica*. Furthermore, Sargeaunt et al. (1980a) proved that *E. histolytica*-like organisms have patterns similar to *E. moshkovskii,* and that both of them are different from *E. histolytica*. *E. invadens* and *E. chattoni* were also characterized by their isoenzyme bands.

More recently, Sargeaunt et al. (1980b) have conducted a pilot survey of a large number of samples collected from hospital patients in Mexico City. A more complex situation emerged than was envisioned in the light of the early results: the invasive strains were no longer concentrated in one group, but three new isoenzyme groups associated with clinical amebiasis were found, as well as four new groups in asymptomatic cyst passers. However, when a total of eleven different isoenzyme groups were studied with respect to the pattern of a single enzyme, hexokinase, only two distinct patterns were distinguished. One was common to patients with clinical amebiasis, and the other was found in patients reported as asymptomatic carriers.

These results have demonstrated the extreme usefulness of isoenzyme studies in differentiating morphologically similar entamoebas. It is disappointing, however that the cultures of *E. histolytica* from cases of invasive amebiasis do not display one, but four different enzymic groups. It appears that more patterns of typical *E. histolytica* will be found as a greater number of specimens are studied from different geographical areas. For this reason, the possible diagnostic value of this technique remains doubtful, but the biological significance of the results in terms of the identification of specific differences between pathogenic and nonpathogenic species of *E. histolytica* is of great interest. However, future studies should better define the status of the "asymptomatic carrier." Only when stringent conditions of negative serology, negative clinical history, and negative rectosigmoidoscopy are obtained in a cyst passer can the case be considered as truly asymptomatic (Sepúlveda and Martínez-Palomo 1982).

An additional taxonomic criterion that may be used to identify different members of the *E. histolytica* group is the analysis of the total protein electrophoretic patterns, proposed recently by Saíd and López-Revilla (1978).

CHAPTER 5
Immunology of Amebiasis*

5.1. Characterization of Amebic Antigens

The characterization of the antigenic components of *E. histolytica* has been one of the main goals of the study of the parasite. Their definition is of relevance both for the improvement of diagnostic methods and for the analysis of the immunological reaction of the infected host, which includes the possibility of inducing protective immunity. In the past, the general tendency was to use aqueous extracts of total antigen, but the present trend is toward the qualitative and quantitative identification of the main antigens of the parasite. Early attempts to characterize the antigenic composition of *E. histolytica* gave poor results because amebas were grown with bacteria from the intestinal tract of man, or in association with other protozoa (Sen et al 1961).

The definition of the immunoelectrophoretic pattern of *E. histolytica* was facilitated by the availability of axenic cultures (Lunde and Diamond 1969) that eliminated foreign antigens from associated organisms. A preliminary characterization of the physicochemical properties of amebic antigens, including the electrophoretic analysis of purified fractions, demonstrated the heterogeneity of the antigenic make-up of the amebas (Alam and Ahmad 1974).

---

*In collaboration with Dr. Bernardo Sepúlveda.

Refinements in the identification of antigens have progressively increased the list of precipitin bands given by crude or fractionated extracts of axenic *E. histolytica* in the presence of homologous antiserum. Krupp (1977) identified fourteen antigens from axenically cultured *E. histolytica* that reacted with sera patients from different geographical locations. She reported that the patterns were basically similar, with minor strain differences being interpreted as due to variations in the relative amount of the antigenic components of the ameba. Another source of difference may be the prolonged culture of *E. histolytica* over several years, perhaps resulting in the disappearance or masking of certain antigens (Bos 1978). The marked increase in resolution provided by double immunoelectrophoresis was exploited by Chang et al.(1979) who obtained up to thirty-two precipitin peaks from axenic strains of *E. histolytica*. These studies have shown that different strains of amebas have a large number of antigens in common, particularly those that induce a humoral antibody response in infected human beings. Recently, Sawhney et al. (1980) partially purified a soluble glycoprotein antigen with hemagglutinating and precipitating properties similar to those described in crude extracts from axenic amebas.

The detection of *E. histolytica* antigen in the serum of patients with invasive amebiasis is of particular importance. It could probably allow a more accurate assessment of the infectious process than does the detection of antibodies. This antigen was found in a few patients in a preliminary study (Ruíz-Castañeda et al. 1976). Using counterimmunoelectrophoresis, Mahajan and Ganguly (1980) have detected amebic antigen in the necrotic material of 92 % of the cases of human liver abscess included in their study.

Circulating antigen-antibody complexes have not been found in patients with amebic liver abscesses (Ortiz-Ortiz et al 1974). This fact was confirmed by Meerovitch et al (1978).

Recently, *E. histolytica* antigens have been detected in feces with the ELISA method (Palacios et al. 1978). In general, this method reveals a higher number of positive cases than the direct microscopic examination of feces. Although further experience is required for the evaluation of the sensitivity and specificity of this method, it seems promising, particularly when the ever-present problem of the correct identification of intestinal protozoa in feces is considered.

5.2 Subcellular Location of Amebic Antigens

The amebic antigen in human infections was initially considered to chiefly originate from a "microsomal" fraction after disruption of the organisms (Boonpucknavig 1967). McLaughlin and Meerovitch (1975a) supported the view that the significant antigens are located in the cytoplasm of the amebas, associated with vesicles that are probably of a lysosomal nature. Recently, purified antigens have been obtained from *E. histolytica* lysosomal and ribosomal fractions (Arroyo-Begovich 1978).

Other evidence indicates that antiamebic antibodies are also produced against surface antigens. O'Shea and Feria-Velasco (1974) using immunofluorescence and immunoelectron microscopy found that purified IgG of sera from patients with active amebiasis binds to the surface of axenically cultured trophozoites of *E. histolytica*. Following our demonstration of the rapid polar redistribution of surface components of *E. histolytica* trophozoites induced by interaction with ligands (Pinto da Silva et al. 1975; Trissl et al. 1977; Martínez-Palomo et al. 1980b), Calderón et al. (1980) demonstrated that fluorescent human antibodies induce a capping phenomenon on the trophozoite surface.

Because the turnover between the surface and internal membranes appears to be particularly rapid in *E. histolytica* trophozoites, antigenic determinants may be located in the recycling cytoplasmic and plasma membranes. This would explain the effective immunogenicity of lysosomal and ribosomal fractions and the location of antigenic components on the surface of the parasite. The chemical composition of the *E. histolytica* plasma membrane is complex since at least twelve glycoproteins can be identified in isolated plasma membrane fractions (Aley et al 1980).

5.3 Humoral Immune Reactions

The humoral immune reaction both in human and experimental invasive amebiasis is mainly characterized by the prompt appearance of specific circulating antibodies. Counterimmunoelectrophoresis (CIE) (Sepúlveda et al 1971, 1972) and indirect hemagglutination (IHA) (Sepúlveda 1970) are the most specific and sensitive tests for these antibodies. Both methods have been reported to coincide in both positive and negative results in more than 90 % of the cases (Sepúlveda 1976) (Table 2); this figure has been confirmed by other workers (Krupp 1974a; Kairalla et al 1976; de Bonilla et al 1978).

TABLE 2

SEROLOGIC REACTIONS IN AMEBIASIS. COMPARISON OF RESULTS EMPLOYING INDIRECT HEMAGGLUTINATION (IHA) AND COUNTER-IMMUNOELECTROPHORESIS (CIE)

	Number	Percentage of positive reactions	
		IHA	CIE
PERSONS WITHOUT EVIDENCE OF AMEBIASIS	224	5.8	6.0
ASYMPTOMATIC CARRIER OF E. HISTOLYTICA	30	6.6	6.6
PATIENTS WITH AMEBIC ABSCESS OF THE LIVER	228	94.8	96.4

Most antiamebic antibodies in the sera of patients with amebic liver abscesses belong to the immunoglobulin G (IgG) class (Maddison et al. 1968; Lee et al. 1970), probably corresponding to IgG subclass 2 since they are not heterocytotropic in guinea pig ileum. As far as other immunoglobulins are concerned, the levels of IgA are frequently elevated in the serum of patients with amebic liver abscesses, although to a lesser extent than those of IgG (Perches et al. 1970). The lack of homocytotropic antibodies was demonstrated by Arellano and Ortiz-Ortiz (1974), suggesting that specific IgE is not present.

It has been shown that immune serum and antiamebic gammaglobulin produce lysis of 90 % of *E. histolytica* trophozoites (Chévez et al. 1973; Sepúlveda et al. 1973a). This lytic effect is suppressed by adsorption of the serum or gammaglobulin with amebas or with crude amebic antigen (Sepúlveda et al 1974a). Furthermore, immune serum neutralizes the virulence of pathogenic *E. histolytica* in culture (Sepúlveda et al. 1974b).

The complement system is another humoral factor involved in the defense against *E. histolytica*. Fresh serum without detectable antiamebic antibodies can induce lysis of approximately 49% of the cell population when used in a 1:3 dilution. Lysis under these conditions has been shown to be a complement-dependent process activated by the alternative pathway (Ortiz-Ortiz et al. 1978; Huldt et al. 1979). In addition, recent studies have shown that hamsters treated with cobra venom factor, which depletes complement, had a higher frequency and severity of hepatic lesions after challenge with virulent amebas (Capín et al. 1980).

The identification of circulating antibodies is of great importance for the diagnosis of invasive amebiasis, and particularly for the detection of the frequent cases that present atypical manifestations. In cases of amebic liver abscess and other severe forms of *E. histolytica* infection, the frequency of positive reaction usually exceeds 95%. On the other hand, in persons without evidence of amebiasis and in carriers, the frequency of positive reactions remains below 10%. Antibodies remain for several months or years after successful treatment. Both hemagglutinins and precipitins may persist for a period of 1 to 5 years (Krupp and Powell 1971; Healy et al. 1974). These facts should be taken into consideration in the interpretation of serological results, since a positive reaction may reflect a previous rather than a present infection. The intensity of the serological reaction has no correlation with the severity of infection.

5.4 Possible Means of Evasion of the Humoral Immune Response

Despite natural and immune defenses, amebas may survive in tissues, multiply, and give rise to invasive amebiasis. Living trophozoites of pathogenic *E. histolytica* strains may well be endowed with mechanisms that allow the survival of the parasite confronted with the immune response of the host. One possible mechanism is capping, or the surface redistribution of membrane antigens in amebas, suggested to be a way of circumventing the effect of specific antibodies bound to the surface (Trissl et al. 1977; Aust-Kettis and Sundqvist 1978). Calderón et al.(1980) have found that antiamebic antibodies bind to *Entamoeba* and induce a redistribution of surface components toward the uroid. The surface segregation results in the accumulation of folded membranes that extrude as a cap containing most of the antibodies that were originally bound to the surface. The cap is subsequently released, probably by the constriction of a limiting connecting region. Further studies into the nature of the released cap are quite feasible since caps can be isolated from living amebas by mechanical agitation (Trissl et al. 1976).

The dynamic nature of the cell surface of *E. histolytica* is also reflected in the release of surface molecules into the extracellular environment. A pronounced shedding of surface components is induced by the incubation of living trophozoites with high concentrations of ligands (Martínez-Palomo and Trissl, unpublished results). The significance of this phenomenon remains to be interpreted. In addition, the development of resistance to complement-mediated immune lysis may occur in cultures of pathogenic *E. histolytica* (Calderón and Tovar-Gallegos 1980).

5.5 Cellular Immune Reactions

The cell-mediated immune response in amebiasis has been studied in vivo using the delayed hypersensitivity skin test. In vitro studies have mainly concentrated on the detection of lymphocyte mitogenic factors and the macrophage inhibitory factor (MIF). Early results obtained following the intradermal injection of amebic antigen did not show a clear-cut correlation with serological findings (Maddison et al 1968; Miller et al 1973; Savanat et al 1973a). This discrepancy could be due to variations in the antigen used and to differences in the time of reading the skin reactions. In addition, skin tests were performed on patients from whom precise information about the clinical stage of the disease was lacking, i.e., time of onset of symptoms, and differentiation between carriers and cases of invasive amebiasis.

With the standardized antigen preparations from axenic cultures of *E. histolytica* and a more accurate evaluation of clinical conditions, a large proportion of patients with active amebic liver abscesses did not give a positive skin response (Kretschmer et al 1972). However, the skin test was negative only for the amebic antigen. Other antigens such as streptokinase and streptodornase produced a positive reaction, indicating that the transient immunosuppression was of a specific nature (Ortiz-Ortiz et al 1975). The number of circulating T cells, as assayed by the T rosette technique, was normal in these patients. During the initial phases of amebic liver abscess only a few patients gave a positive skin response. The skin reactions became positive in the majority of patients one month after clinical recovery (Ortiz-Ortiz et al. 1975; Landa et al. 1976).

Lymphocytic transformation rates induced by concanavalin A in patients with amebic liver abscesses do not significantly differ from those in normal individuals, although slightly lower values were found in the former group (Ortiz-Ortiz et al. 1975). Similar results were reported by Harris and Bray (1976) using phytohemagglutinin to induce lymphocyte activation in leukocytes from patients with amebiasis. Recently, Gold et al. (1978) have found a lowered reactivity of hamster lymphocytes to phytohemagglutinin and concanavalin A in experimentally infected animals.

In general, the MIF test gave results similar to those obtained with the skin test in cases of human invasive amebiasis (Ortiz-Ortiz et al. 1975). Results were generally negative during the initial phases of liver infection and became positive after treatment of the hepatic abscess. Specific antibodies were found at the beginning and during the subsequent stages of the disease in patients with negative intradermal and MIF reactions. In experimental amebiasis, the cellular immune response was also depressed during the initial phases of induced liver abscess (Ortiz-Ortiz et al. 1973; Gold et al. 1978). Under such conditions, the serological reactions were positive.

Even if the above mentioned tests seem to indicate that the primary immune response in amebiasis is predominantly humoral, it is evident that cell-mediated immunity participates in some way from the beginning of the infectious process. It has been shown that the administration of immunosuppressive drugs favors the development of experimentally induced amebic hepatic abscesses in hamsters (Tanimoto-Weki et al. 1974). In addition, only mice immunosuppressed with antilymphocytic serum develop liver lesions after intracecal inoculation of virulent amebas (Wijesundera 1980). On the other hand, aqueous extracts of *E. histolytica* (Savanat et al. 1973b) or a subcellular antigenic fraction of *E. histolytica* composed mainly of lysosomal membranes (Segovia et al. 1980) induces blastogenic transformation of lymphocytes from patients with amebic liver abscesses, suggesting the sensitization of T lymphocytes to amebic antigens. Recently, Diamantstein et al. (1980) have reported the mitogenic activity of *E. histolytica* extracts on murine lymphocytes.

5.6 Resistance to Reinfection

Following the elimination of amebic infection in dogs, it was shown that 83% of the animals were completely refractory to reinfection by either homologous or heterologous strains of *E. histolytica*, and the resistance to infection probably persisted longer than nine months (Swartzwelder and Avant 1952). Similar results were obtained in adult hamsters; after successful treatment of experimental amebic liver abscess, 70% of the animals were refractory to the intrahepatic reinoculation of virulent amebas (Vázquez-Saavedra et al.1973).

In human beings, recurrence of liver abscess after successful treatment is extremely rare, occurring in only 0.29% of 1021 patients followed for five years (de León 1970). In severe forms of amebic colitis, recurrence is also exceptional. Even in benign amebic dysentery, true recurrence with characteristic clinical and endoscopic findings and isolation of hematophagous *E. histolytica* trophozoites from lesions is uncommon, notwithstanding the fact that patients continue to live in a highly contaminated environment. Consequently, on the basis of clinical evidence it appears that partial or complete resistance can be acquired by human beings after recovery from amebic infection.

5.7 Induction of Protective Immunity

The induction of protective immunity against intrahepatic inoculation of virulent amebas was demonstrated in adult hamsters using crude axenic antigen from *E. histolytica* or live trophozoites (Sepúlveda et al. 1973b; Tanimoto-Weki et al. 1973). Partial protection, probably passive immunity, was also achieved in hamsters with human immune serum (Sepúlveda et al. 1974b). Subsequently, it was shown that ribosomal and lysosomal antigenic fractions isolated from axenic *E. histolytica* induced protective immunity against intrahepatic inoculation of virulent amebas in suckling hamsters. These purified fractions exhibited stronger antigenic properties in vitro and in vivo than did the crude amebic antigen used previously (Sepúlveda et al. 1978).

The above mentioned results were corroborated in adult hamsters which were protected against intrahepatic challenge after intradermal injection of living trophozoites (Ghadirian and Meerovitch 1978). Protective immunity was also induced in guinea pigs by an antigenic high molecular weight fraction isolated from axenic *E. histolytica*. The animals did not develop cecal lesions following direct inoculation of virulent amebas (Krupp 1974b; Vinayak et al. 1980).

CHAPTER 6
Parasite Factors of Virulence

One of the fundamental questions of the biology of *E. histolytica* directly related to the understanding of human amebiasis concerns the nature of the factors that determine the virulence of the parasite and the switch from a harmless commensal to an aggressive invader. The initiation of invasive amebiasis results from the rupture of the host-parasite equilibrium that is maintained while *E. histolytica* is restricted to the commensal phase. This imbalance leads to an alteration in the normal life cycle of the parasite, since invasive amebas enter into a phase biologically deleterious for their survival in which cyst production ceases. It is evident that the rupture of the balance between parasite and host may be produced by changes in either or both participants; however, the nature of these changes is less obvious. Among a variety of possible host factors, consideration has been given to geographical location, race, sex, age, nutritional and immunological status, diet, local climate, and sexual habits. Clinical experience has indicated that the most frequent severe form of invasive amebiasis, i.e., liver abscess, occurs in certain geographical areas where virulent strains of *E. histolytica* are prevalent. They affect mostly adult males living under conditions of crowding, poverty, and ignorance that favor repeated infection through fecalism due to inadequate disposal of human excreta and improper food handling. No specific host factors other than those conducive to constant exposure to virulent strains of amebas have been shown to play a decisive role in the establishment of intestinal or liver lesions in those countries in which invasive amebiasis represents a common and important health problem. The following review will mainly concentrate on parasite virulence factors, the main focus of the majority of recent investigations.

6.1 Virulence of Pathogenic Strains

The term pathogenicity is used to denote the general ability of an organism to produce disease, whereas virulence refers to that ability, but under certain specified conditions that imply degree (Gladstone 1970).

The relative degree of virulence of a given strain of *E. histolytica* may significantly vary during prolonged culture with mixed bacterial populations. However, the intrinsic virulence of a strain grown under axenic conditions in a given experimental model remains basically the same. While axenic strains of high virulence consistently are able to produce liver abscesses in newborn hamsters over a period of several years, strains of attenuated virulence require much higher inocula to produce the same effect. Axenic cultures of isolates from well-characterized human asymptomatic carriers and cultures of low-temperature *Entamoeba* fail to demonstrate pathogenicity over the same length of time, when similar culture conditions and assays of pathogenicity are used.

Taking into account the relatively stable pathogenicity of axenic cultures, a number of properties have been compared in strains of differing virulence with the aim of understanding the cellular basis of pathogenicity in *E. histolytica* (Trissl et al. 1977, 1978; Martínez-Palomo et al. 1980b; Orozco et al. 1980). The results are shown in Table 3.

TABLE 3
SURFACE PROPERTIES OF VARIOUS STRAINS OF E. HISTOLYTICA

Property	Pathogenic Strains	Nonpathogenic Strains
IN VITRO CYTOPATHIC EFFECT	++++	0
RATE OF ERYTHROPHAGOCYTOSIS	++++	+
AGGLUTINATION WITH CON A	++++	+
SURFACE BINDING OF CON A	++++	+
NEGATIVE SURFACE CHARGE	0 - +	+
ADHESION TO EPITHELIAL CULTURES	++	++
RATE OF CAP FORMATION	++++	++++

Two of the cell surface properties that clearly separate pathogenic from nonpathogenic strains of *E. histolytica* are the rate of erythophagocytosis and the extent of contact-dependent cytopathic effects measured in vitro. Both properties are directly correlated with the degree of in vivo virulence of various pathogenic strains of the parasite cultured under axenic conditions.

Among a variety of surface properties tested, the agglutination induced by the plant lectin concanavalin A, which clumps cells when mannose- or glucose-containing residues are located free on the surface of the cell, clearly distinguishes the strains isolated from cases of human dysentery and those obtained from asymptomatic carriers (Martínez-Palomo et al. 1973). The former are more susceptible to lectin-induced agglutination because they have a much higher number of exposed surface receptors, demonstrated by immunofluorescence (Trissl et al. 1978) and surface labeling with iodinated concanavalin A (Martínez-Palomo and Calderón, unpublished data).

6.2 Viruses and Virulence

The presence of various types of viruses or virus-like particles in trophozoites of *E. histolytica* has been documented by electron microscopy in amebas obtained from human lesions, and by a number of biological assays in strains cultured under axenic conditions, as reviewed in sections 2.2.5 and 2.2.6. Rhabdovirus-like, filamentous, and polyhedral viruses have been found, but efforts to infect animals or cultured cells, as well as attempts to demonstrate their presumptive role as vehicles for the transfer of episome-like virulence factors have failed (Bird and McCaul 1976; Diamond and Mattern 1976). Axenic cultures of *E. histolytica* show no acquisition of pathogenicity that could be ascribed to the replication of a lysogenic virus capable of inducing the transformation of commensal trophozoites into invasive cells able to destroy tissues and resist the natural defenses of the host. Considering the extremely rudimentary state of knowledge of the cellular genetics of pathogenic protozoa in general, and of *E. histolytica* in particular, only a strong development of this field will enable these potentially fascinating hypotheses to be proved. At present, they cannot be explored due to our frustrating ignorance of certain aspects of the biology of the parasite.

6.3 Virulence and Culture Conditions

The virulence of pathogenic strains of *E. histolytica* may vary with the following culture conditions: a) association with mixed bacterial flora, specific bacteria (e.g., *Fusobacterium symbiosus*), or a protozoan (*Trypanosoma cruzi*); b) number of subcultures; c) periodic passage and reculture from liver lesions of experimental animals; and d) addition of cholesterol to the culture medium.

6.3.1. Bacterial associates

The dogmatic assertion that *E. histolytica* is unable to express its pathogenic capability unless grown in association with bacteria prevailed for several decades in spite of repeated demonstrations that amebas produce liver necrosis in man usually in the absence of association with other microorganisms, since liver abscesses in humans are generally sterile. The cultivation of *E. histolytica* under axenic conditions (Diamond 1968) was met with interest by those concerned with the biochemistry of the parasite, but initially received little attention from experimental parasitologists, some of whom considered axenic cultures of *E. histolytica* as a sort of in vivo aberration having little in common with the amebas that destroy epithelial tissue in man. This idea was strengthened by the results of Phillips et al (1972) who reported the failure of axenic strains to produce invasive amebic lesions in germ-free guinea pigs, in contrast to the production of lesions by cultures grown in association with bacteria.

The addition of bacterial flora from isolates of differing degrees of invasiveness or the addition of pathogenic bacteria to cultures did not significantly alter the virulence of amebic strains (Neal 1957). However, separation of the trophozoites from associated intestinal flora induced a rapid decline in virulence over a period of weeks or months (Bos and Hage 1975), while reassociation with bacteria over a number of subcultures was reported to result in the reacquisition of pathogenicity. Under the conditions used by Wittner and Rosenbaum (1970), *E. histolytica* had to be associated with nonpathogenic living bacteria for more than 6 hours in order to become pathogenic and produce liver lesions after direct inoculation in hamsters or guinea pigs. Bacterial extracts or killed bacteria had no effect. These observations suggested the possibility that the virulence of *E. histolytica* could depend on an episome-like factor that required direct contact with bacteria in order to be expressed. Mixed and, in some instances, monoxenic cultures of amebas are still needed to consistently produce intestinal ulcerations in experimental animals, mainly guinea pigs and rats. Axenic cultures of pathogenic strains of *E. histolytica* are able to erode the cecal mucosa of conventionally raised newborn guinea pigs (Diamond et al. 1978b) and hamsters (Ghadirian and Meerovitch 1979), but variations in the strain of guinea pig and/or cecal microflora hinder the uniform production of intestinal lesions by axenic strains.

The role of bacteria in the establishment of *E. histolytica* colonies and subsequent invasion of the colonic mucosa in experimental models is far from being understood. On the one hand, bacteria may hinder the direct contact and attachment of trophozoites to the apical surface of epithelial intestinal cells by the formation of a continuous layer covering the mucosa of the large intestine. For this reason, the production of amebic lesions is more reproducible when animals are treated with laxatives or antibiotics before trophozoites are introduced into the intestinal lumen. On the other hand, bacteria may provide directly, or indirectly through the breakdown of extracellular components, certain nutrients, including iron, necessary for the vigorous growth of the amebas in the intestine. The transmission by bacteria of an episome-like agent that would transform amebas into invasive cells remains, as previously mentioned, an unproven hypothesis.

There is substantial evidence that axenic pathogenic cultures of *E. histolytica* can produce liver lesions in hamsters. The first conclusive demonstration was made by Tanimoto et al. (1971) who directly injected large numbers of amebas into the liver to produce liver abscesses in adult hamsters. The important finding that *E. histolytica* cultured without bacterial associates can produce liver necrosis was corroborated by various authors (Diamond et al. 1974a; Martínez-Palomo 1978; Ghadirian and Meerovitch 1979; Lushbaugh et al. 1981). The greater susceptibility of newborn hamsters to developing liver lesions following the inoculation of virulent amebas was demonstrated by Mattern and Keister (1977). In this experimental model, an inoculum of only a few amebas is sufficient to produce focal hepatic necrosis. These lesions lead to a progressive necrosis of the liver and death in approximately 3 weeks (Lushbaugh et al. 1980b; Martínez-Palomo et al. 1980c). Production of liver lesions in adult hamsters requires increasingly larger inocula with age. In adult animals, inoculation of amebas through the portal vein results in the formation of multiple liver abscesses. A natural susceptibility, similar to the hamster, to develop liver lesions when trophozoites are injected is also found in the gerbil (Diamond et al. 1974b). In contrast, mice and guinea pigs are not susceptible under similar conditions.

6.3.2 Cholesterol

Cholesterol is required for the growth of *E. histolytica* in culture. The observation of an increase in the virulence of trophozoites following the addition of cholesterol to the culture (Sharma 1959) was succeeded by reports on the facilitation of experimentally induced invasive amebiasis in guinea pigs fed with cholesterol (Biagi et al. 1963; Gargouri 1967). More recently, a new wave of interest in the effects of cholesterol on the pathogenicity of *E. histolytica* has resulted from reports that the virulence of cultured amebas that have lost their pathogenicity can be restored by cholesterol (Das and Ghoshal 1976; Bos and van de Griend 1977; Meerovitch and Ghadirian 1978). The restoration of virulence of axenic strains appears to require from 10 to 20 passages in the presence of cholesterol. An alteration of the lipid composition of amebic membranes might somehow be related to an increase in virulence. However, this possibility can be ruled out because even though the membrane lipid composition may vary to a certain extent according to the nature of the exogenously supplied lipids, the virulence of the trophozoites persists even after cholesterol is removed. An alternative explanation is that since cholesterol is added in particulated form, the procedure may select for those amebas that have a higher phagocytic index, and probably a high level of virulence.

6.3.3 Number of passages in culture

Prolonged cultivation of *E. histolytica* with mixed bacterial flora has generally been considered to invariably result in loss of virulence (Neal 1957). In contrast, axenic cultures of pathogenic strains undergo only small changes, expressed as a relative increase or decrease in virulence (Diamond et al. 1974a; Ghadirian and Meerovitch 1979; de la Torre, Tanimoto, and Martínez-Palomo, unpublished observations). Serial passage of amebic cultures through experimental animals has been known to increase the virulence of xenic cultures; this procedure also alters the virulence of axenic trophozoites (Lushbaugh et al. 1978).

6.3.4. Strain heterogeneity

One possible explanation of the differences in the virulence of cultivated pathogenic strains of *E. histolytica* is that each strain is composed of a heterogeneous mixture of genetically unrelated substrains, each one with a different degree of virulence. Certain favor the selective growth of the less virulent substrains, whereas other experimental procedures such as serial passage through the liver or the administration of particulated cholesterol would result in the selection of those substrains with higher phagocytic capacity and virulence. In fact, selection of poorly phagocytic amebas from the highly virulent and phagocytic strain HM1:IMSS through treatment with poisonous bacteria has resulted in the isolation of a substrain of attenuated virulence (Orozco, Guarneros, and Martínez Palomo, unpublished observations). This finding indicates the existence of a certain amount of heterogeneity in strains of axenically cultivated *E. histolytica*. Nevertheless, strains do not appear to be very heterogeneous, since a number of clones isolated from the strain HM1:IMSS differ very little from the wild strain (Orozco and Martínez-Palomo, unpublished observations).

It appears that alterations in the virulence of cultured axenic strains of *E. histolytica* are more likely to be the consequence of selective pressure rather than the result of an induced transformation state that leads to a change from a nonpathogenic to a pathogenic condition. The main virulence factors are intrinsic to the amebas and are probably modulated by culture conditions. Thus, virulence is not exclusively triggered by the association of *E. histolytica* with bacteria, as has traditionally been thought to be the case.

6.4 Attachment

Similar to many other microorganisms that colonize and invade the epithelia, *E. histolytica* can adhere to the surface of a variety of mammalian cells: epithelial cells, erythrocytes, leukocytes, macrophages, etc. In spite of the evidence accumulated during recent years on the importance of the attachment phase for the expression of virulence in certain enteropathogenic bacteria, very little is known about the attachment of *E. histolytica* to target cells, and its role, if any, in the initiation of invasive amebiasis. Trophozoites probably do not attach to the intestinal epithelium during the commensal phase of *E. histolytica*, being separated from the plasma membrane of epithelial cells of the lining by the surface coat of microvilli, bacterial flora, mucus, and debris. The infrequent finding of amebas attached to the intestinal epithelium may also be explained by the fact that the apical surfaces of epithelial cells are normally less adhesive than the free surfaces of other cell types. Attachment of amebas to the free surface of the intestinal mucosa is only rarely found in biopsy specimens in early invasive intestinal amebiasis (Prathap and Gilman 1970). As discussed below, the penetration of amebas into the mucosal wall is initially limited to the interglandular regions, possibly because amebas preferentially adhere to the surface of desquamating cells, and subsequently find weak pathways for invasion in these regions. In other zones of the intestinal mucosa, viable cells are bound to each other by occluding junctions and are covered by a thick surface coat that may hinder the adhesion of trophozoites.

Electron microscopy has shown that trophozoites of *E. histolytica* may establish close contact with mammalian cells in vitro, leaving an intercellular space approximately 20 nm in width between the adjoining plasma membranes. In addition to the electrostatic interactions and chemical bonds established between the exposed molecules of the converging surfaces, adhesion depends on the active metabolism of the amebas, since the trophozoites form an ectoplasmic band of fibrogranular material, possibly actin microfilaments, at the site of attachment. Attachment is reduced by low temperatures, cell poisoning, and by the action of the microfilament depolymerizing drug cytochalasin B.

Probably relevant for the understanding of the initial phases of invasive intestinal amebiasis is the question of whether variations in the degree of adherence to epithelial surfaces exist between strains of differing virulence. Recent studies have demonstrated that the rate of adhesion of several strains of *E. histolytica* to different mammalian cell surfaces is similar, regardless of the relative degree of virulence shown by each strain (Orozco, Martinez-Palomo, and Mora, unpublished observations). In a microscopic study of the cytopathic effect of *E. histolytica* on cultured epithelial cells combining microcinematography, transmission, and scanning electron microscopy, we have observed that attachment is the first phase in a series of reactions leading to the killing of target cells. Interference with attachment will block the cytotoxic activity of the amebas. Therefore, it has become evident that attachment, although necessary for the expression of the pathogenicity of *E. histolytica*, does not vary in strains exhibiting differing degrees of virulence. A lectin from axenically grown *E. histolytica* trophozoites has been isolated and partially characterized by Kobiler and Mirelman (1980). This lectin agglutinates different types of erythrocytes and may be involved in the adherence of amebas to host cells.

The scanning electron microscope has revealed some possible ways of blocking the attachment of *E. histolytica* to the apical surface of intestinal cells - the first step in the invasion of the intestinal wall. The cecal mucosa in conventionally raised guinea pigs is frequently covered by a carpet of bacteria tightly adhering to the epithelium, thus establishing a living barrier between the amebas and the mucosal surface. Under these conditions, eradication of the bacteria with antibiotics prior to the inoculation of the amebas considerably increases the possibility of adhesion and penetration of the trophozoites through the mucosal surface. This observation shows that, at least in some experimental models, the colonization of the intestinal surface with certain bacteria may reduce the possibility of amebic infection and penetration by interfering with attachment (Mora Galindo, González-Robles and Martínez -Palomo, unpublished observations).

6.5 Multiplication and Penetration

The ability to grow in vivo is another virulence factor in invasive microorganisms. Growth is determined by the nutritional requirements of the parasite and the ability of the host environment to provide these nutrients. The establishment of lumenal amebiasis involves the multiplication of *E. histolytica* in the commensal phase, the colonization of certain regions of the colon, and the formation of cysts. These activities require adequate conditions for parasite survival that probably include a specific bacterial flora. The conditions that determine the switch from the commensal phase to the invasive phase of *E. histolytica* are essentially unknown. This particular aspect of the host-parasite interaction represents the most important challenge for research on the pathogenesis of invasive amebiasis. The understanding of the factors that favor this change necessitates knowledge of the mechanisms by which trophozoites rupture the intestinal barriers of natural immunity and overcome local reactions of induced humoral and cellular immunity. The role of metal ions and particularly the requirements for iron in amebiasis may be important for the outcome of the host-parasite relationship since free iron is usually not available to invading microorganisms, which must compete for it.

In spite of their striking lytic ability, trophozoites of *E. histolytica* do not seem to easily penetrate the intact intestinal mucosa. Careful examination of biopsies from early cases of human intestinal lesions have suggested that amebas penetrate the intact epithelium of the large intestine only in the interglandular regions (Prathap and Gilman 1970). In experimental in vivo and in vitro models in which the interaction between trophozoites and the cecal mucosa of the guinea pig was analyzed, the initial penetration of amebas was limited to the interglandular regions (Mora et al. 1978) (Figures 48 and 49). These represent areas of low resistance where dying cells are continuously being sloughed off as the final step in the unceasing renewal of the mucosal lining. By attachment and preferential phagocytosis of desquamating cells, trophozoites accumulate at the interglandular zones and penetrate by means of active movement and phagocytosis into the deeper mucosal layers where they proliferate. Therefore, it can be expected that conditions that promote the desquamation of intestinal epithelial cells favor the development of invasive intestinal amebiasis. The fact that amebas find a more suitable environment for multiplication and lytic activity in the subepithelial layers is clearly revealed by the

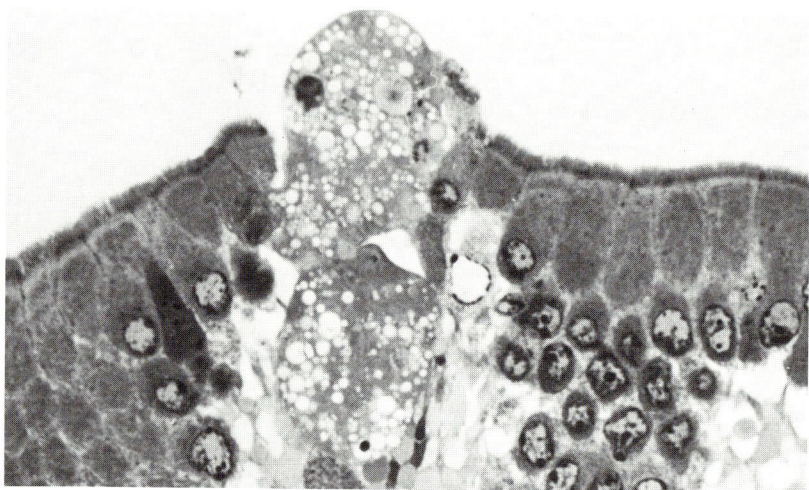

Figure 48. Light micrograph of the surface of the guinea pig cecal epithelium. Two amebas have penetrated through the intercellular space. X 850.

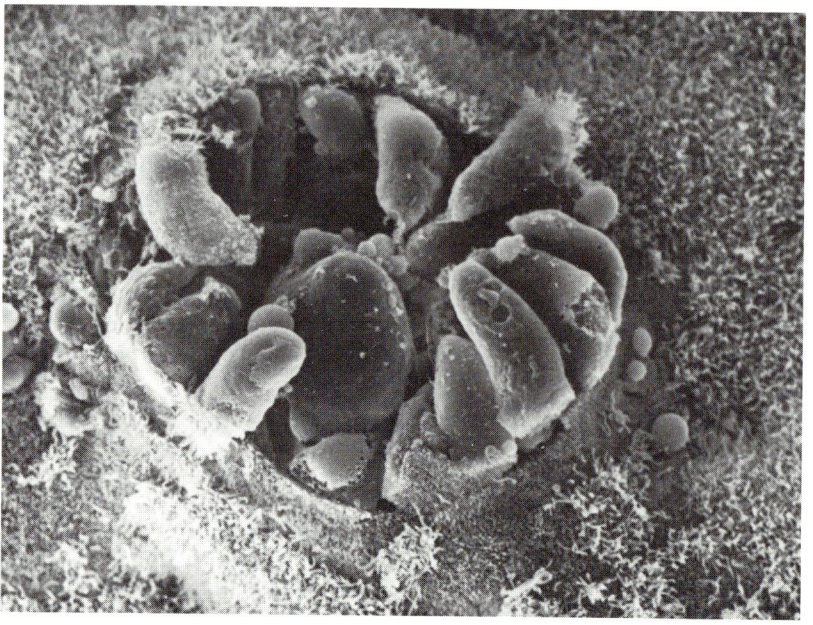

Figure 49. Scanning electron micrograph of a microulceration of the cecal epithelium. X 1,000.

classic bottleneck appearance of small amebic ulcers, consisting of a small opening at the epithelial lining and a large basal region of destruction in the deeper mucosal layers where most of the amebas are found.

Once trophozoites have breached the natural barriers of the intestinal epithelium, the striking motility of the parasite facilitates its passage through the mucosa. The invasive capacity of *E. histolytica* is also due to its scavenging ability, combining the lysis and phagocytosis of mammalian cells. The secretion of lytic enzymes as a means of parasite dissemination has been investigated by several groups. Collagenase activity was initially detected by the action of trophozoites on gelatin (Jarumilinta and Maegraith 1969), and more recently has been analyzed in detail by Muñoz et al. (1982).

Hyaluronidase and proteolytic activities have been reported in extracts of *E. histolytica*, but their significance remains doubtful since they are equally present in pathogenic and nonpathogenic amebas (Jarumilinta and Maegraith 1969). Even though the battery of amebic enzymes capable of hydrolyzing mammalian tissues has yet to be completely analyzed, clinical evidence gives a clear indication of their potency and variety, since many human tissues, including skin, bone, and cartilage, can be destroyed by *E. histolytica*.

6.6 Evasion of Host Defenses

The ability of *E. histolytica* to survive and damage its host depends, in addition to the previously discussed factors, on the ability of the parasite to abolish or reduce the effectiveness of the natural and acquired host defenses. Resistance to complement may be one of the mechanisms by which *E. histolytica* survives during invasive infections. Trophozoites pretreated with antibodies are resistant to the effect of antibodies plus human complement (Calderón and Tovar-Gallegos 1980). Furthermore, the ligand-induced redistribution of surface antigens or capping (Pinto da Silva et al.1975; Trissl et al.1978; Calderón et al.1980), followed by the shedding of plasma membrane antigens bound to antibodies may be a mechanism that allows *E. histolytica* trophozoites to evade the humoral immune response of the host. In addition, a substantial quantity of the redistributed antibodies may be internalized (Aust-Kettis and Sundqvist 1980), and a certain proportion of the rapid loss of antibodies from the surface of the amebas may be due to their dissociation from antigenic determinants (Aust-Kettis et al. 1981). The possible resistance of trophozoites to other molecules that act extracellularly, such as basic polypeptides and lysozymes, has not been studied.

The in vitro interaction between *E. histolytica* and white blood cells or macrophages usually results in the killing of mammalian cells, unless a ratio of more than several hundred cells to one ameba is used (Guerrant et al.1981). Significantly, trophozoites of a highly virulent strain were not killed even when each ameba was confronted with 3,000 human polymorphonuclear leukocytes, whereas a strain of attenuated virulence was susceptible to these cells (Guerrant et al.1981). This result suggests that resistance to leukocyte killing may be a virulence determinant in *E. histolytica*. Further studies are needed to determine whether virulent strains are more resistant to macrophage cytotoxicity and phagocytosis.

6.7 Cytotoxicity

The analysis of the parasite factors that bring about the killing of host cells is one of the most intensely studied subjects in experimental amebiasis. The powerful lytic activity of the parasite, described in its name, has inspired a variety of approaches aimed at understanding the biological basis of this phenomenon. One of the main drawbacks of most of these studies is that only a single factor has been considered, e.g., aggression by a specific organelle, a toxin, or an enzyme. It is clear that the cytopathic effect of *E. histolytica* on mammalian tissues cannot be attributed to a single action on the part of the parasite and that the scavenging activity of the ameba is the combined result of various chemical and mechanical mechanisms.

Time-lapse microcinematography has been of considerable value in the in vitro analysis of the mechanisms of host cell damage induced by *E. histolytica*. Studies of trophozoites confronted with white blood cells (Chévez and Segura 1974; Guerrant et al. 1981), fibroblasts (Ravdin et al. 1980), or with various types of epithelial cells (Chévez et al. 1976; Martínez-Palomo and Cervantes, unpublished observations) have convincingly demonstrated the importance of movement-dependent processes as a means of parasite aggression. Contact between amebas and target cells may be followed by strong attachment and the displacement of cells from their original positions through the active motility of the trophozoites. Amebas may produce small phagocytic stomas that incorporate minute portions of the periphery of target cells, followed by abrupt separation, resulting in the rupture of the plasma membrane and subsequent lysis of the host cell. This mechanism of "pinching off" the cell membrane has also been demonstrated in the killing of tumor cells by macrophages (Chambers and Weiser 1969).

6.7.1 Toxins in homogenates of trophozoites

There is no laboratory or clinical evidence that pathogenic strains of *E. histolytica* produce substances similar to the potent exotoxins of certain bacteria (i.e., botulin toxin, tetanus toxin, diphtheria toxin). In contrast, sonicates of *E. histolytica* have consistently been shown to have components that are toxic for mammalian red blood cells. The existence of a degrading mechanism for human red blood cells in *E. histolytica* is obvious, since virulent trophozoites avidly ingest and degrade red blood cells. Erythrocytes provide a simple system to test the lytic properties of amebic extracts, and have been used for many years to demonstrate cytolysis produced by *E. histolytica* (Craig 1927; Vinayak and Chitkara 1976; López-Revilla and Saíd-Fernández 1980). The chemical nature of the hemolysin, its location in the ameba, and its significance, if any, in the cytopathogenic mechanisms of *E. histolytica* remain to be determined.

In contrast with the results obtained with red blood cells, attempts to demonstrate cytopathic effects of *E. histolytica* sonicates on nucleated mammalian cells were unsuccessful for many years because amebic proteins with cytotoxic activity are inhibited by components in the serum. Different groups simultaneously obtained, concentrated, partially purified, and assayed the cytotoxic activity of intracellular amebic toxins (Bos 1979; Lushbaugh et al. 1979; Mattern et al. 1980). Cytotoxic activity is restricted to proteins ranging in molecular weight from 25,000 to 35,000 daltons, and can be found at protein concentrations as low as 2–4 μg/ml (Lushbaugh et al. 1979). Even though the cytotoxin has enterotoxic activity, demonstrated by the induction of fluid secretion in ligated rabbit ileal loops, the pathogenic role of the toxin remains uncertain. Cytotoxicity assays using cultured cells have only revealed a rounding-up of the cells followed by their release from the substrate. This reaction indicates that the amebal toxin produces retraction and detachment of the cells, but has no effect on their viability (Ravdin et al. 1980). Furthermore, there is no evidence that this toxin is released by amebas during the cytotoxic reaction. The activity of the toxin becomes apparent after up to 24 hours of incubation with cultured cells, whereas living trophozoites of a virulent strain will completely lyse and digest a monolayer of epithelial cells in approximately one hour when present in a 1:1 ratio (Orozco et al. 1978). However, there are differences in the cytotoxic activity of amebic sonicates obtained from strains of varying virulence (Lushbaugh et al. 1980a). Based on the characteristics of the serum inhibition of the amebic toxin, Lushbaugh et al. (1981) have suggested that the toxin has protease activity.

6.7.2 Contact-dependent cytopathic effect

Attempts to understand the cytopathogenic mechanisms of *E. histolytica* using animal models have generally involved the morphological analysis of intestinal or liver lesions days or weeks after inoculation of the amebas. With these models it has been possible to demonstrate that the interglandular regions of the cecal mucosa are the initial sites of penetration of the amebas (Mora et al. 1978), and that during the early stages of liver abscess formation, a pronounced granulomatous inflammatory reaction occurs (Aguirre-García et al. 1972; Martínez-Palomo 1978; Lushbaugh et al. 1980b). However, the details of the interaction between amebas and host cells that leads to the killing of the latter in a matter of seconds or minutes can only be analyzed using in vitro systems in which the process can be followed by microcinematography and by various forms of light and electron microscopy, and the interaction can be experimentally modified.

Three main cellular systems have been used for in vitro studies of amebic cytotoxicity: leukocytes, fibroblasts, and epithelial cells. Red blood cells are rapidly engulfed by the trophozoites of pathogenic strains of *E. histolytica* through a process of agglutination, attachment, phagocytosis in which the shape of the red blood cells is considerably distorted, and intracellular degradation (Trissl et al. 1978). There is no evidence that the erythrocyte membrane is altered by the action of an amebic hemolysin before red blood cells are ingested by trophozoites.

Leukocyte suspensions were one of the first systems used in the microscopic study of amebic cytopathogenicity. Both the protozoan parasite and the host white blood cells are able to kill each other. However, unless the leukocyte to ameba ratio is very large, virulent amebas are able to kill phagocytes. The most important observation derived from the use of this model is that direct contact between the ameba and the cell membrane is required in order to kill the target cell (Jarumilinta and Kradolfer 1964; Artigas et al. 1966; Bos 1973; Chévez et al. 1976; Guerrant et al. 1981). When confronted with amebas of low virulence in a favorable ratio, polymorphonuclear leukocytes kill the amebas, apparently through anaerobic mechanisms (Guerrant et al. 1981). The way in which amebas kill leukocytes remains unknown, except for the fact that direct contact is required and that killing is followed by ingestion. Kinetic studies of the interaction between *E. histolytica* and leukocytes are difficult to interpret because both cell types can kill each other, and lysis may be due not only to the cytotoxic action of the opponent cell, but also to the liberation of lytic enzymes from dying cells of both types. In addition, the time between contact, adhesion, and lysis varies considerably.

Killing of polymorphonuclear leukocytes by *E. histolytica* has been shown to occur in vivo both in human intestinal lesions (Griffin 1972) and in early stages of hepatic abscess formation in young hamsters (Martínez-Palomo, unpublished observations).

A recent analysis of the interaction between virulent *E. histolytica* and Chinese hamster ovary cells (CHO) has clearly demonstrated that amebic cytopathogenicity has two stages: a contact-dependent cytolethal phase, followed by phagocytosis of the lysed cells (Ravdin et al 1980). Cultured CHO cells not in contact with the amebas remain viable, while practically all the target cells are killed before phagocytosis.

Morphological observations of the contact-dependent cytopathic effect of *E. histolytica* initially suggested that the parasite was endowed with a "trigger-like" organelle, the so-called surface-active lysosome, that "fired" upon contact with host cells, liberating lytic enzymes and thus initiating lysis (Eaton et al 1969, 1970). The idea of a protozoan pathogen equipped with a microscopic weapon ready to be discharged when confronted with mammalian cells attracted much attention, but this hypothesis has not been validated. Surface lysosomes are equally present in pathogenic and nonpathogenic *Entamoeba*, and no evidence for their participation in contact cytolysis has been found using microcinematography or electron microscopy (see section 2.3.6).

The lysis of cultured epithelial cells by *E. histolytica* also begins by contact, followed by selective membrane damage and osmotic swelling of the host cells. The latter has been suggested to be due to the action of a membrane-like phospholipase (Knight et al 1975; McCaul 1977; McCaul and Bird 1977; McCaul et al 1977).

Most of the observations made by Ravdin et al (1980) and McCaul and Bird (1977) have been confirmed with the use of an in vitro system in which the interaction between epithelial monolayers in culture and pathogenic amebas can be studied (Orozco et al 1978; Orozco et al 1980). The morphological and functional properties of this cultured epithelium from the MDCK cell line have been extensively characterized (Cereijido et al 1980; Martínez-Palomo et al 1980a). MDCK monolayers provide a suitable model because they consist of a single even sheet of tightly adhering cells that form a continuous layer resembling the epithelial barrier faced by *E. histolytica* in vivo. After contact between a trophozoite and the apical surface of the epithelial monolayer is established (Figure 50), the ameba spreads over the target cells and may produce distortion and the disappearance of surface microvilli (Figure 51). The first sign of cellular damage demonstrable by microcinematography and electron microscopy is the widening of the intercellular spaces due to the opening of the occluding junctions along the upper margin of the lateral borders of the cells. The gap between adjacent cells increases in width due to a sizeable retraction of the cells in different regions of the monolayer. In certain cells, a portion of the periphery may be pinched off by the amebas (Figure 52), followed by the formation of large cytoplasmic blebs and subsequent lysis of the damaged cells. However, the most frequently observed phenomenon is the formation of multiple membranous blebs after amebas have been in contact with the free surface of epithelial cells for periods ranging from a few seconds to several minutes. The damaged cells are mechanically dislodged by moving trophozoites (Figure 53), and are finally phagocytized in various stages of lysis (Figure 54). The last step involves the intracellular degradation of the engulfed cells (Figures 55).

The mechanism through which trophozoites exert the contact-dependent cytotoxicity that precedes the formation of surface blebs and lysis has not yet been determined. Although ultrastructural evidence of membrane fusion between cytoplasmic vacuoles and the inner face of the plasma membrane of the amebas has been obtained, no proof of a true exocytosis of lytic components, or of the existence of a membrane-bound toxin that would act upon contact with target cells has been found.

Our knowledge of the cellular mechanisms of ameba cytotoxicity is at a level comparable to that concerning the cytotoxicity of T lymphocytes and macrophages. All three require living effector cells that act through intimate contact with and firm adhesion to target cells, leading to plasma membrane damage. In subsequent stages, phagocytosis plays an important role in both macrophage and ameba-induced cytotoxicity through the incorporation of whole lysed cells or the pinching off of portions of the target cell surface. In all three systems, damage may be produced in the target cell membrane through a membrane-bound enzyme or the liberation of a cytolytic product acting at a short distance. Why killer cells do not get destroyed during the lytic process and whether or not an exocytic mechanism is involved are questions that remain unresolved in terms of macrophage (Chambers and Weiser 1969; Sharma and Piessens 1978; Key and Haskill 1981), T lymphocyte (Allison and Ferluga 1975; Biberfeld and Johansson 1975; Sanderson 1976;

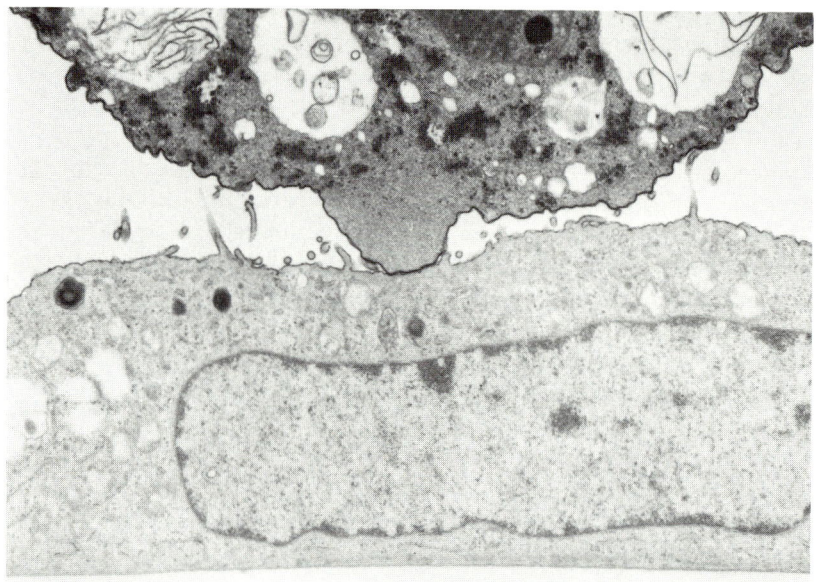

Figure 50. Contact between the pseudopodium of an ameba and a MDCK cell in culture. X 8,000.

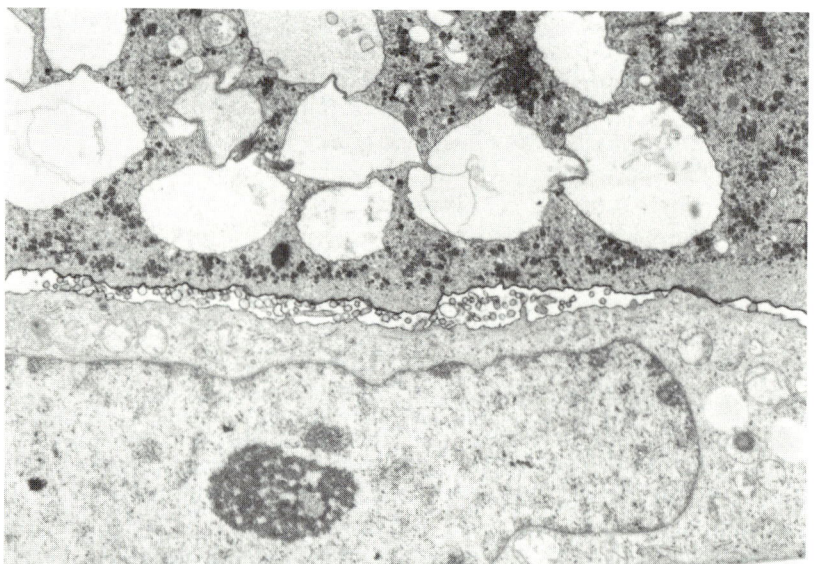

Figure 51. Close contact between an ameba and a MDCK cell. Epithelial microvilli are collapsed. X 8,000.

115

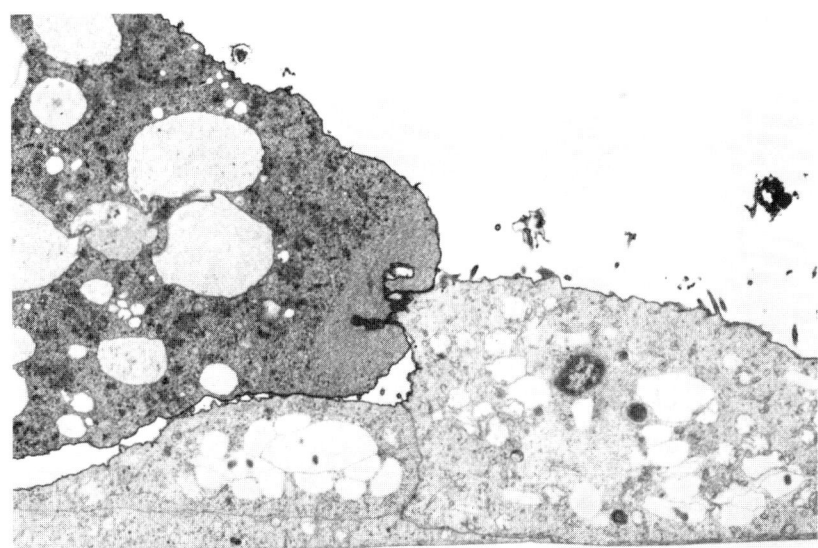

Figure 52. Pinching off of the cytoplasm of a cultured epithelial cell by a trophozoite. X 8,000.

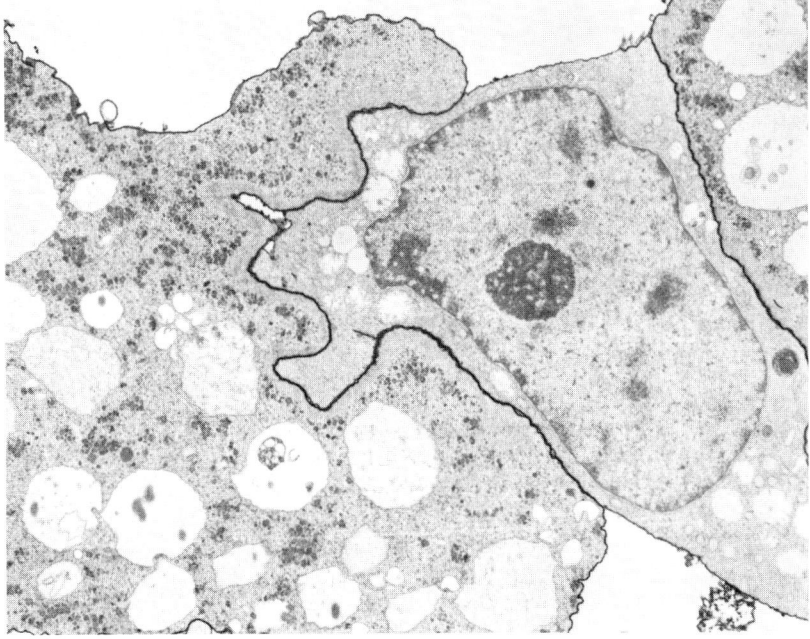

Figure 53. Two trophozoites displace an epithelial cell from the culture substrate. X 8,000.

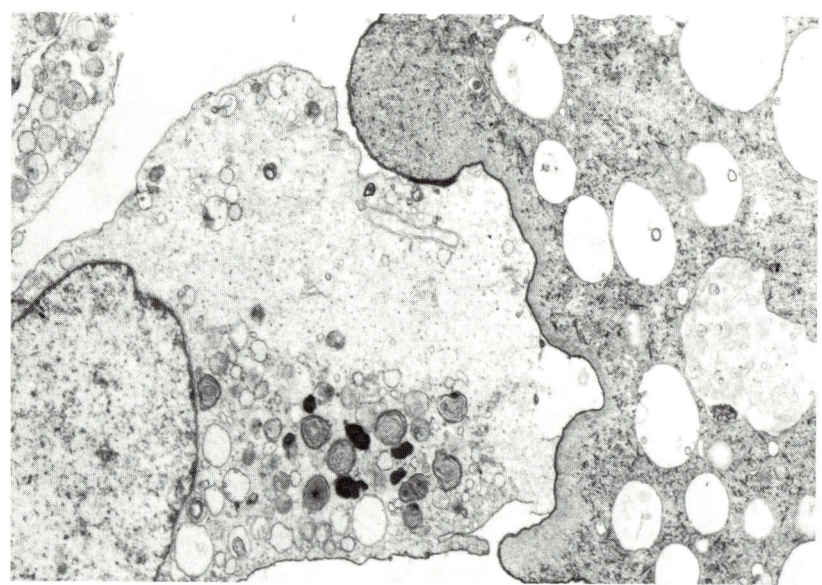

Figure 54. Phagocytosis of a lysed epithelial cell by a trophozoite. X 8,000.

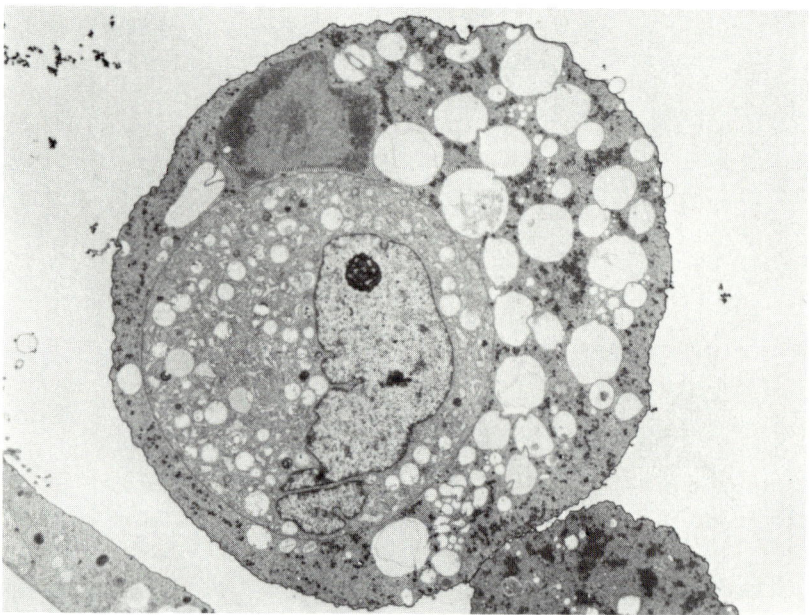

Figure 55. Intracellular degradation of an epithelial cell phagocytosed by an ameba. X 8,000.

Henney 1977), and ameba-induced cytotoxicity.

It can be concluded that the cytotoxic action of *E. histolytica* requires the activity of living trophozoites of pathogenic strains and the establishment of close contact with the target cells. Damage of mammalian cells by the amebas is achieved through a combination of mechanical and chemical means, the latter probably involving a membrane-bound toxin that produces osmotic damage in the plasma membrane of target cells. Lysis is followed by ingestion of the damaged cells by means of phagocytosis. Finally, degradation of phagocytized cellular components within the phagocytic vacuoles of the amebas completes the killing action of *E. histolytica*.

The in vitro cytotoxic mechanisms previously described may be operative in vivo, although this remains to be demonstrated. In intestinal and liver amebic lesions, necrosis may also be the result of the death and disintegration of amebas (Villarejos 1962) and inflammatory cells (Griffin 1972). During the early stages of experimental amebic abscess, the liberation of lytic enzymes by numerous macrophages could also contribute to the spread of the necrosis (Martínez-Palomo 1978).

CHAPTER 7
Some Unsolved Problems in Amebiasis Related to the Biology of the Parasite

A review of the available information concerning the biology of *E. histolytica* described in previous chapters has pointed out the existence of a number of unanswered questions relevant for the understanding of human amebiasis. The following is a partial summary of these problems.

Differentiation between pathogenic and nonpathogenic species of E. histolytica: The future characterization and rapid axenization of invasive and noninvasive strains, together with the use of techniques in the fields of biochemical taxonomy and cellular cytogenetics, will probably resolve the problem of whether different species of *Entamoeba* are responsible for the worldwide distribution of lumenal amebiasis and the geographically more restricted occurrence of invasive amebiasis. Details on the mechanism of nuclear division in both types of strains may reveal as yet undetected biological differences which could eventually serve as the basis for the design of simple and reliable diagnostic procedures to characterize pathogenic *E. histolytica*. Such an advance would annually spare millions of people from the unnecessary and possibly harmful effects of amebicidal drugs by restricting treatment to those harboring pathogenic strains of *E. histolytica*.

Identification of the mechanisms underlying the transformation from the commensal to the invasive state: The search for parasite and host factors responsible for the triggering of the invasive capacity of trophozoites must be continued. This is the most crucial and least understood aspect of the pathogenesis of the disease.

Cyst differentiation: The design of axenic media that permit the differentiation of trophozoites into cysts would considerably facilitate the study of the biochemical aspects of encystation and excystation. Prevention of either of these two phases through interference with enzyme reactions not found in the host could eventually lead to the development of potent cysticides lacking toxicity towards man. The interruption of the life cycle of the parasite could, in principle, provide a biological alternative for the prophylaxis of the disease.

Characterization of amebic products responsible for cytotoxicity: Since there is no indication that the toxin obtained from amebic lysates participates in the killing of host cells, further studies are needed in order to characterize what appears to be a membrane-bound toxin, and to determine whether it is delivered to the target cell through exocytosis or other mechanisms.

Characterization of amebic antigens: The identification of those antigenic components of the ameba that are relevant in terms of the humoral immune response, and the mass production of these antigens through monoclonal antibodies produced by hybridomas could provide the basis for better diagnostic methods of invasive amebiasis.

Protective immunity: The importance of this issue has been emphasized by the clinical finding that invasive amebiasis rarely occurs in the same patient twice, and by the experimental induction of protective immunity in mammals. The characterization of pure and potent antigens with the aid of monoclonal antibodies produced by hybridomas could be of considerable value in this respect.

Design of new amebicides: Drugs presently available for the treatment of invasive amebiasis, such as dehydroemetine and metronidazole, produce numerous side effects. In addition, the known cardiac and neurologic toxicity of emetine and the potential cancerigenic activity of metronidazole should prompt the development of equally effective but harmless drugs to treat invasive amebiasis, possibly taking advantage of the recent advances in knowledge of the biochemistry of the parasite.

Pathogenesis: The early stages of amebic invasion in the large intestine and the liver remain to be analyzed, both in man and in experimental models. The extent, nature, and role of the inflammatory reaction during different stages of liver abscess in man remain a mystery. Another important and unsettled aspect of the pathology of human amebiasis, probably linked to a parasite factor, is the lack of deposition of fibrous tissue following treatment of invasive lesions; destructive intestinal, hepatic, and even skin lesions usually heal with complete anatomical restitution after successful treatment. The question of whether the local multiplication of fibroblasts and the deposition of fibrous tissue are inhibited during the healing process have yet to be answered.

CHAPTER 8
References

Aguirre-García, J., Calderón, P. and Tanimoto-Weki, M. (1972). Examen histopatológico de las lesiones hepáticas en hamsters inoculados con cultivo axénico de *Entamoeba histolytica*. Archivos de Investigación Médica (Mexico), 3, Suppl. 2, 341-348.

Alam, M. and Ahmad, S. (1974). Immunogenicity of *Entamoeba histolytica* antigen fractions. Transactions of the Royal Society of Tropical Medicine and Hygiene, 68, 370-373.

Albach, R.A., Shaffer, J.G. and Watson, R.H. (1966). A comparison of in vitro drug sensitivities of strains of *Entamoeba* which grow at 37°C and at room temperature. American Journal of Tropical Medicine and Hygiene, 15, 855-859.

Albach, R.A., Booden, T., Boonlayangoor, P. and Downing, S. (1980). Concepts of function of peripheral non-chromatin and endosome in *Entamoeba histolytica*. Archivos de Investigación Médica (Mexico), 11, Suppl. 1, 63-74.

Aley, S.B., Scott, W.A. and Cohn, Z.A. (1980). Plasma membrane of *Entamoeba histolytica*. Journal of Experimental Medicine, 152, 391-404.

Allison, A.C. and Feruluga, J. (1976). How lymphocytes kill tumor cells. New England Journal of Medicine, 295, 165-167.

Anonymous. (1979). Pathogenic *Entamoeba histolytica*. Lancet, 1, 303.

Arellano, M.T. and Ortiz-Ortiz, L. (1974). Algunas propiedades de la globulina específica del suero de pacientes con absceso hepático amibiano. Archivos de Investigación Médica (Mexico), 5, Suppl. 2, 487-490.

Arroyo-Begovich, A. (1978). Inducción de inmunidad protectora antiamibiana con "nuevos" antígenos en el hamster lactante. B. Material antigénico. Archivos de Investigación Médica (Mexico), 9, Suppl. 1, 311-314.

Arroyo-Begovich, A., Cárabez-Trejo, A. and Ruíz-Herrera, J. (1980). Identification of the structural component in the cyst wall of *Entamoeba invadens*. Journal of Parasitology, 66, 735-741.

Artigas, J., Otto, I. and Kawada, M.E. (1966). Acción de *Entamoeba histolytica* sobre leucocitos polimorfonucleares humanos vivos. Boletín Chileno de Parasitología, 21, 114-118.

Aust-Kettis, A. and Sundqvist, K.G. (1978). Dynamics of the interaction between *Entamoeba histolytica* and components of the immune response. I. Capping and endocytosis: Influence of inhibiting and accelerating factors; variation of the expression of surface antigens. Scandinavian Journal of Immunology, 7, 35-44.

Aust-Kettis, A. and Sundqvist, K.G. (1980). Dynamics of the interaction between *Entamoeba histolytica* and components of the immune response. II. On the distinction of surface bound and internalized anti-amoeba antibodies. Scandinavian Journal of Immunology, 12, 443-451.

Aust-Kettis, A., Lidman, K. and Fagraeus, A. (1977). Actin in *Entamoeba histolytica* trophozoites revealed by human actin antibodies. Journal of Parasitology, 63, 581-583.

Aust-Kettis, A., Thorstensson, R. and Sundqvist, K.G. (1981). Dynamics of the interaction between *Entamoeba histolytica* and components of the immune response. III. Fate of antibodies after binding to the cell surface. Scandinavian Journal of Immunology, 13, 473-481.

Bailey, G.B. and Rengpien, S. (1980). Osmotic stress as a factor controlling encystation of *Entamoeba invadens*. Archivos de Investigación Médica (México) 11, Suppl. 1, 11-16.

Balamuth, W. (1962). Effects of some environmental factors upon growth and encystation of *Entamoeba invadens*. Journal of Parasitology, 48, 101-109.

Band, R.N. and Cirrito, H. (1979). Growth response of axenic *Entamoeba histolytica* to hydrogen, carbon dioxide, and oxygen. Journal of Protozoology, 26, 282-286.

Barker, D.C. and Deutsch, K. (1958). The chromatoid body of *Entamoeba invadens*. Experimental Cell Research, 15, 604-610.

Barker, D.C. and Svihla, G. (1964). Localization of cytoplasmic nucleic acid during growth and encystment of *Entamoeba invadens*. Journal of Cell Biology, 20, 389-398.

Barker, D.C. and Swales, L.S. (1972a). Characteristics of ribosomes during differentiation from trophozoite to cyst in axenic *Entamoeba* sp. Cell Differentiation, 1, 297-306.

Barker, D.C. and Swales, L.S. (1972b). Comparison of trophozoite helical polysomes with cyst ribosomogen microcrystals in axenic *Entamoeba* sp. Cell Differentiation, 1, 307-315.

Barry, J.D. (1979). Capping of variable antigen on *Trypanosoma brucei*, and its immunological and biological significance. Journal of Cell Science, 37, 287-302.

Bernhard, W. and Avrameas, S. (1971). Ultrastructural visualization of cellular carbohydrate components by means of concanavalin A. Experimental Cell Research, 64, 232-236.

Biagi, F.F., Robledo, E., Servín, H. and Martuscelli, A. (1962). The effect of cholesterol on the pathogenicity of *Entamoeba histolytica*. American Journal of Tropical Medicine and Hygiene, 11, 333-340.

Biberfeld, P. and Johansson, A. (1975). Contact areas of cytotoxic lymphocytes and target cells. An electron microscope study. Experimental Cell Research, 94, 79-87.

Bird, R.G. and McCaul, T.F. (1976). The rhabdoviruses of *Entamoeba histolytica* and *Entamoeba invadens*. Annals of Tropical Medicine and Parasitology, 70, 81-93.

Boonlayangoor, P., Albach, R.A., Stern, M.L. and Booden, T. (1978). Entamoeba histolytica: Uptake of purine bases and nucleosides during axenic growth. Experimental Parasitology, 45, 225-233.

Boonpucknavig, S., Lynraven, G.S., Nairn, R.C. and Ward, H.A. (1967). Subcellular localization of Entamoeba histolytica antigen. Nature, 216, 1232-1233.

Bos, H. (1973). The problem of pathogenicity in parasitic Entamoeba. Acta Leidensia, 40, 1-112.

Bos, H.J. (1975). Monoxenic and axenic cultivation of carrier and patient strains of Entamoeba histolytica. Zeitschrift für Parasitenkunde, 47, 119-129.

Bos, H.J. (1978). Fractionation and serological characterization of Entamoeba histolytica antigen. Acta Leidensia, 45, 105-116.

Bos, H. (1979). Entamoeba histolytica: Cytopathogenicity of intact amebae and cell-free extracts: Isolation and characterization of an intracellular toxin. Experimental Parasitology, 47, 369-377.

Bos, H.J. and Hage, A.J. (1975). Virulence of bacteria-associated, crithidia-associated, and axenic Entamoeba histolytica: Experimental hamster liver infections with strains from patients and carriers. Zeitschrift für Parasitenkunde, 47, 79-89.

Bos, H.J. and van de Griend, R.J. (1977). Virulence and toxicity of axenic Entamoeba histolytica. Nature, 265, 341-343.

Bowers, B. and Korn, E.D. (1968). The fine structure of Acanthamoeba castellani. I. The trophozoite. Journal of Cell Biology, 39, 95-111.

Brumpt, E. (1925). Étude sommaire de l' "Entamoeba dispar" n.sp. Amibe à kystes quadrinucléés, parasite de l'homme. Bulletin de l'Académie de Médecine (Paris), 94, 943-952.

Brumpt, E. (1949). Précis de Parasitologie, pp. 183-224. Masson, Paris.

Burrows, R.R. (1957). Entamoeba hartmanni. American Journal of Hygiene, 65, 172-188.

Calderón, J. and Tovar-Gallegos, G.R. (1980). Resistance to immune lysis induced by antibodies in *Entamoeba histolytica*. In The Host-Invader Interplay, Ed. H. Van den Bossche, pp. 227-230. Elsevier/North Holland, Amsterdam.

Calderón, J., Muñoz, M.L. and Acosta, H.M. (1980). Surface redistribution and release of antibody-induced caps in *Entamoebae*. Journal of Experimental Medicine, 151, 184-193.

Capín, R., Capín, N.R., Carmona, M. and Ortiz-Ortiz, L. (1980). Effect of complement depletion on the induction of amebic liver abscess in the hamster. Archivos de Investigación Médica (Mexico), 11, Suppl. 1, 173-180.

Cerbón, J. and Flores, J. (1981). Phospholipid composition and turnover of pathogenic amebas. Comparative Biochemistry and Physiology, 69B, 487-492.

Cereijido, M., Ehrenfeld, J., Martínez-Palomo, A. and Meza, I. (1980). Structural and functional membrane polarity in cultured monolayers of MDCK cells. Journal of Membrane Biology, 52, 147-160.

Cervantes, A. and Martínez-Palomo, A. (1980). Estudio del ciclo vital de *Entamoeba invadens* mediante cinematografía espaciada. Archivos de Investigación Médica (Mexico), 11, Suppl. 1, 31-40.

Chambers, V.C. and Weiser, R.S. (1969). The ultrastructure of target cells and immune macrophages during their interaction in vitro. Cancer Research, 29, 301-317.

Chang, S.M., Lin, C.M., Dusanic, D.G. and Cross, J.H. (1979). Antigenic analyses of two axenized strains of *Entamoeba histolytica* by two-dimensional immunoelectrophoresis. American Journal of Tropical Medicine and Hygiene, 28, 845-853.

Charoenlarp, P., Reeves, R.E. and Warren, L.G. (1968). Carbohydrate utilization by *Entamoeba histolytica*. Experimental Parasitology, 23, 205-211.

Chávez, B., Martínez-Palomo, A. and de la Torre, M. (1978). Estructura ultramicroscópica de la pared de quistes de *Entamoeba invadens, E. histolytica* y *E. coli*. Archivos de Investigación Médica (Mexico), 9, Suppl. 1, 113-116.

Chévez, A. and Segura, M. (1974). Interacción entre los trofozoítos de *E. histolytica* y los leucocitos de varias especies animales. Archivos de Investigación Médica (Mexico), 5, Suppl. 2, 373-382.

Chévez, A., Segura, M., Iturbe, I. and Aubanel, M. (1971). Aspectos morfológicos en la biología del trofozoíto de *Entamoeba histolytica* desde el punto de vista de la citología dinámica. Archivos de Investigación Médica (Mexico), 2, Suppl. 1, 229-244.

Chévez, A., Corona, D., Segura, M. and Iturbe-Alessio, I. (1972a). La pinocitosis como expresión anabólica de *Entamoeba histolytica*. Archivos de Investigación Médica (Mexico), 3, Suppl. 2, 265-274.

Chévez, A., Iturbe-Alessio, I., Segura, M. and Corona, D. (1972b). Fagocitosis de eritrocitos humanos por *Entamoeba histolytica*. Archivos de Investigación Médica (Mexico), 3, Suppl. 2, 275-286.

Chévez, A., Iturbe-Alessio, I., Sepúlveda, B., Segura, M. and Ortíz-Ortíz, L. (1973). Respuesta morfodinámica de los trofozoítos de *E. histolytica* a la acción del suero humano inmune correspondiente. Archivos de Investigación Médica (Mexico), 4, Suppl. 1, 71-78.

Chévez, A., Sepúlveda, B., Segura, M., Corona, D. and Díaz, J. (1976). Initial phases of pathogenic activity of *E. histolytica* in colon and liver of hamster. *In* Proceedings of the International Conference on Amebiasis, Ed. B. Sepúlveda and L.S. Diamond, pp. 420-517. Instituto Mexicano del Seguro Social, Mexico City.

Cleveland, L.R. and Sanders, E.P. (1930). Encystation, multiple fission without encystment, excystation, metacystic development and variation in a pure line and nine strains of *Entamoeba histolytica*. Archiv für Protistenkunde, 70, 15-261.

Coleman, J.R., Nilsson, J.R., Warner, R.R. and Batt, P. (1973). Effects of calcium and strontium on divalent ion content of refractive granules in *Tetrahymena pyriformis*. Experimental Cell Research, 80, 1-9.

Councilman, W.T. and Lafleur, H.A. (1891). Amoebic dysentery. Johns Hopkins Hospital Reports, 2, 395-548.

Craig, C.F. (1927). Observations upon the hemolytic, cytolytic and complement-binding properties of extracts of *Endamoeba histolytica*. American Journal of Tropical Medicine, 7, 225-240.

Czeto, A.R., Morgan, R.S. and Strother, G.K. (1973). The ultraviolet absorption spectra of chromatoid bodies of *Entamoeba invadens* in situ. Experimental Cell Research, 78, 345-350.

D'Antoni, J.S. (1952). Concepts and misconceptions in amebiasis. American Journal of Tropical Medicine, 1, 146-154.

Das, S.R. and Ghoshal, S. (1976). Restoration of virulence to rat of axenically grown *Entamoeba histolytica* by cholesterol and hamster liver passage. Annals of Tropical Medicine and Parasitology, 70, 439-443.

Deas, J.E. and Miller, J.H. (1977). Plasmalemmal modifications of *Entamoeba histolytica* in vivo. Journal of Parasitology, 63, 25-31.

de Bonilla, L., Healy, G.R., Scott, F. and Visvesvara, G.V. (1978). Reproducibility of indirect hemagglutination and countercurrent electrophoresis tests on sera from patients in an area of endemic amebiasis. Archivos de Investigación Médica (Mexico), 9, Suppl. 1, 349-350.

de Carneri, I. (1959). The use of specific anti-amoebic drugs for comparative taxonomic studies. Transactions of the Royal Society of Tropical Medicine and Hygiene, 53, 120-121.

de León, A. (1970). Pronóstico tardío en el absceso hepático amibiano. Archivos de Investigación Médica (Mexico), 1, Suppl., s205-s206.

Deschiens, R. (1965). L'Amibiase et l'Amibe Dysentérique. Masson, Paris.

Deutsch, K. and Zaman, V. (1959). An electron microscopic study of *Entamoeba invadens* Rodhain 1934. Experimental Cell Research, 17, 310-319.

Diamantstein, T., Trissl, D., Klos, M., Gold, D. and Hanh, H. (1980). Mitogenicity of *Entamoeba histolytica* extracts for murine lymphocytes. Immunology, 41, 347-352.

Diamond, L.S. (1961). Axenic cultivation of *Entamoeba histolytica*. Science, 134, 336-337.

Diamond, L.S. (1968). Techniques of axenic cultivation of *Entamoeba histolytica* Schaudinn, 1903, and *E. histolytica*-like amebae. Journal of Parasitology, 54, 1047-1056.

Diamond, L.S. (1980). Axenic cultivation of *Entamoeba histolytica*: Progress and problems. Archivos de Investigación Médica (Mexico), 11, Suppl. 1, 47-54.

Diamond, L.S. and Mattern, C.F.T. (1976). Protozoal viruses. Advances in Virus Research, 20, 87-112.

Diamond, L.S., Mattern, C.F. and Bartgis, I.L. (1972). Viruses of *Entamoeba histolytica*. I. Identification of transmissible virus-like agents. Journal of Virology, 9, 326-341.

Diamond, L.S., Phillips, B.P. and Bartgis, I.L. (1974a). A comparison of the virulence of nine strains of axenically cultivated *E. histolytica* in hamster liver. Archivos de Investigación Médica (Mexico), 5, Suppl. 2, 423-426.

Diamond, L.S., Phillips, B.P. and Bartgis, I.L. (1974b). The clawed jird (*Meriones unguiculatus*) as an experimental animal for the study of hepatic amebiasis. Archivos de Investigación Médica (Mexico), 5, Suppl. 2, 465-470.

Diamond, L.S., Harlow, D.R. and Cunnick, C.C. (1978a). A new medium for the axenic cultivation of *Entamoeba histolytica* and other *Entamoeba*. Transactions of the Royal Society of Tropical Medicine and Hygiene, 72, 431-432.

Diamond, L.S., Tanimoto-Weki, M. and Martínez-Palomo, A. (1978b). Production of cecal lesions in newborn guinea pigs with axenically cultivated *Entamoeba histolytica*. Archivos de Investigación Médica (Mexico), 9, Suppl. 1, 223-228.

Dobell, C. (1919). The Amoebae Living in Man. A Zoological Monograph. John Bale, Sons & Danielsson, London.

Dobell, C. (1928). Researches on the intestinal protozoa of monkeys and man. I. General introduction. II. Description of the whole life-history of *Entamoeba histolytica* in cultures.

Parasitology, 20, 357-412.

Dobell, C. (1931). Researches on the intestinal protozoa of monkeys and man. IV. An experimental study of the *histolytica*-like species of *Entamoeba* living naturally in macaques. Parasitology, 23, 1-72.

Doyle, J.J., Behin, R., Mauel, J. and Rowe, D.S. (1974). Antibody-induced movement of membrane components of *Leishmania enriettii*. Journal of Experimental Medicine, 139, 1061-1069.

Eaton, R.D.P., Meerovitch, E. and Costerton, J.W. (1969). A surface-active lysosome in *Entamoeba histolytica*. Transactions of the Royal Society of Tropical Medicine and Hygiene, 63, 678-680.

Eaton, R.D.P., Meerovitch, E. and Costerton, J.W. (1970). The functional morphology of pathogenicity in *Entamoeba histolytica*. Annals of Tropical Medicine and Parasitology, 64, 299-304.

Edelman, M.H. and Spingarn, C.L. (1977). Cultivation of *Entamoeba histolytica* as a diagnostic procedure: A brief review. Mount Sinai Journal of Medicine, 44, 27-32.

El-Hashimi, W. and Pittman, F. (1970). Ultrastructure of *Entamoeba histolytica* trophozoites obtained from the colon and from in vitro cultures. American Journal of Tropical Medicine and Hygiene, 19, 215-226.

Elsdon-Dew, R. (1968). The epidemiology of amoebiasis. Advances in Parasitology, 6, 1-62.

Elsdon-Dew, R. (1971). Amebiasis as a world problem. Bulletin of the New York Academy of Medicine, 47, 438-447.

Elsdon-Dew, R. (1979). Pathogenic *Entamoeba histolytica*. Lancet, 1, 1038-1039.

Entner, N., Evans, L.A. and González, C. (1962). Genetics of *Entamoeba histolytica*: Differences in drug sensitivity between Laredo and other strains of *Entamoeba histolytica*. Journal of Protozoology, 9, 466-468.

Faust, E.C., Russell, P.F. and Jung, R.C. (1970). Clinical Parasitology, 8th edition, pp. 141-170. Lea & Febiger, Philadelphia.

Feria-Velasco, A. and Treviño, N. (1972). The ultrastructure of trophozoites of *Entamoeba histolytica* with particular reference to spherical arrangements of osmiophilic cylindrical bodies. Journal of Protozoology, 19, 200-211.

Feria-Velasco, A., Martínez-Zedillo, G., Treviño-García Manzo, N. and Gutiérrez-Pastrana, M.D. (1973). Investigación del ácido siálico en la cubierta exterior de trofozoítos de *E. histolytica*. Estudio bioquímico y citoquímico de alta resolución. Archivos de Investigación Médica (Mexico), 4, Suppl. 1, s33-s38.

Fletcher, K.A., Maegraith, B.G. and Jarumilinta, R. (1962). Electron microscope studies of trophozoites of *Entamoeba histolytica*. Annals of Tropical Medicine and Parasitology, 56, 496-499.

Freedman, L. and Elsdon-Dew, R. (1959). Size as a criterion of species in the human intestinal amebae. American Journal of Tropical Medicine and Hygiene, 8, 327-330.

Gargouri, M. (1967). L'utilisation du cholestérol dans l'amibiase expérimentale du cobaye. Annales de Parasitologie (Paris), 42, 399-402.

Gelderman, A.H., Keister, D.B., Bartgis, I.L. and Diamond, L.S. (1971). Characterization of the deoxyribonucleic acid of representative strains of *Entamoeba histolytica, E. histolytica*-like amebae, and *E. moshkovskii*. Journal of Parasitology, 57, 906-911.

Ghadirian, E. and Meerovitch, E. (1978). Vaccination against hepatic amebiasis in hamsters. Journal of Parasitology, 64, 742-743.

Ghadirian, E. and Meerovitch, E. (1979). Pathogenicity of axenically cultivated *Entamoeba histolytica*, strain 200:NIH, in the hamster. Journal of Parasitology, 65, 768-771.

Gicquaud, C.R. (1979). Étude de l'ultrastructure du noyau et de la mitose de *Entamoeba histolytica*. Biologie Cellulaire, 35, 305-312.

Gillin, F.D. and Diamond, L.S. (1978). Clonal growth of *Entamoeba histolytica* and other species of *Entamoeba* in agar. Journal of Protozoology, 25, 539-543.

Gillin, F.D. and Diamond, L.S. (1980). Attachment and short-term maintenance of motility and viability of *Entamoeba histolytica* in a defined medium. Journal of Protozoology, 27, 220-225.

Gladstone, G.P. (1970). Pathogenicity and virulence of microorganisms. *In* General Pathology, Ed. H.W. Florey. pp. 823-834. W.B. Saunders, Philadelphia.

Gold, D., Norman, L.G., Maddison, S.E. and Kagan, I.G. (1978). Immunologic studies on hamsters infected with *Entamoeba histolytica*. Journal of Parasitology, 64, 866-873.

Goldman, M. (1969). *Entamoeba histolytica*-like amoebae occurring in man. Bulletin of the World Health Organization, 40, 355-364.

Griffin, J.L. (1972). Human amebic dysentery: Electron microscopy of *Entamoeba histolytica* contacting, ingesting and digesting inflammatory cells. American Journal of Tropical Medicine and Hygiene, 21, 895-906.

Griffin, J.L. and Juniper, K. (1971). Ultrastructure of *Entamoeba histolytica* from human amebic dysentery. Archives of Pathology, 21, 271-280.

Guerrant, R.L., Brush, J., Ravdin, J.I., Sullivan, J.A. and Mandell, G.L. (1981). Interaction between *Entamoeba histolytica* and human polymorphonuclear neutrophils. Journal of Infectious Diseases, 143, 83-93.

Gutteridge, W.E. and Coombs, G.H. (1977). Biochemistry of Parasitic Protozoa. The Macmillan Press, London.

Harlow, D.R., Weinbach, E.C. and Diamond, L.S. (1976). Nicotinamide nucleotide transhydrogenase in *Entamoeba histolytica*, a protozoan lacking mitochondria. Comparative Biochemistry and Physiology, 53B, 141-144.

Harris, W.G. and Bray, R.S. (1976). Cellular sensitivity in amoebiasis. Preliminary results of lymphocytic transformation in response to specific antigen and to mitogen in carrier and disease states. Transactions of the Royal Society of Tropical Medicine and Hygiene, 70, 340-343.

Healy, G.R., Visvesvara, G.S. and Kagan, I.G. (1974). Observations on the persistence of antibodies to *E. histolytica*. Archivos de Investigación Médica (Mexico), 5, Suppl. 2, 495-500.

Henley, G.L., Lee, C.M. and Takeuchi, A. (1976). Freeze-etching observations of trophozoites of pathogenic *Entamoeba histolytica*. Zeitschrift für Parasitenkunde, 48, 181-190.

Henney, C.S. (1977). T-cell mediated cytolysis: An overview of some current issues. Contemporary Topics in Immunology, 7, 245-272.

Hoare, C.A. (1952). The commensal phase of *Entamoeba histolytica*. Experimental Parasitology, 1, 411-427.

Hopkins, D.L. and Warner, K.L. (1946). Functional cytology of *Entamoeba histolytica*. Journal of Parasitology, 32, 175-189.

Hruska, J.F., Mattern, C.F.T., Diamond, L.S. and Keister, D.B. (1973). Viruses of *Entamoeba histolytica*. III. Properties of the polyhedral virus of the HB-301 strain. Journal of Virology, 11, 129-136.

Huldt, G., Davies, P., Allison, A.C. and Schorlemmer, H.U. (1979). Interactions between *Entamoeba histolytica* and complement. Nature, 277, 214-216.

Hummeler, K. and Tomassini, N. (1973). Rhaboviruses. *In* Ultrastructure of Animal Viruses and Bacteriophages, Ed. A.J. Dalton and F. Haguenau, pp. 239-251. Academic Press, New York.

Injeyan, H., Huebner, E. and Meerovitch, E. (1979). Studies on a morphologically distinct colchicine-resistant variant of *Entamoeba* sp. Journal of Protozoology, 26, 253-259.

Jarumilinta, R. and Kradolfer, F. (1964). The toxic effect of *Entamoeba histolytica* on leucocytes. Annals of Tropical Medicine and Parasitology, 58, 375-381.

Jarumilinta, R. and Maegraith, B.G. (1969). Enzymes of *Entamoeba histolytica*. Bulletin of the World Health Organization, 41, 269-273.

Kairalla, A.B., Pittman, F.D., Healy, G.R., Lushbaugh, W.B., Hofbauer, A.F. and Pittman, J.C. (1976). Experience with indirect hemagglutination (IHA) and counterimmunoelectrophoretic amebic (CIEP-A) serologies in clinical practice at a southeastern United States university medical center. *In* Proceedings of the International Conference on Amebiasis, Ed. B. Sepúlveda and L.S. Diamond, pp. 712-720. Instituto Mexicano del Seguro Social, Mexico City.

Kartulis, S. (1887). Zur Aetiologie der Leberabscesse. Lebende Dysenterie-Amöben im Eiter der dysenterischen Leberabscesse. Centralblatt für Bakteriologie und Parasitenkunde, 25, 745-748.

Keller, P.M., Morgan, N.H., Morgan, R.S. and Czeto, A.R. (1973). Tubulin in cysts of *Entamoeba invadens*. Journal of Cell Biology, 59, 165a.

Key, M. and Haskill, S. (1981). Macrophage-mediated, antibody-dependent destruction of tumor cells in DBA/2 mice: In vitro identification of an in situ mechanism. Journal of the National Cancer Institute, 66, 103-110.

Knight, R., Bird, R.G. and McCaul, T.F. (1975). Fine structural changes at *Entamoeba histolytica* rabbit kidney cell (RK13) interface. Annals of Tropical Medicine and Parasitology, 69, 197-202.

Kobiler, D. and Mirelman, D. (1980). Lectin activity in *Entamoeba histolytica* trophozoites. Infection and Immunity, 29, 221-225.

Kofoid, C.A. and Swezy, O. (1925). On the number of chromosomes and the type of mitosis in *Endamoeba dysenteriae*. University of California Publications in Zoology, 26, 331-352.

Korn, E.D. (1975). Biochemistry of endocytosis. *In* Biochemistry of Cell Walls and Membranes, Ed. C.F. Fox, pp. 1-26. Butterworths, London.

Kress, Y., Wittner, M. and Rosenbaum, R.M. (1971). Sites of cytoplasmic ribonucleoprotein-filament assembly in relation to helical body formation in axenic trophozoites of *Entamoeba histolytica*. Journal of Cell Biology, 49, 773-784.

Kretschmer, R.R., Sepúlveda, B., Almazán, A. and Gamboa, F. (1972). Intradermal reactions to an antigen (histolyticin) obtained from axenically cultivated *Entamoeba histolytica*. Tropical and Geographical Medicine, 24, 275-281.

Krishna Murti, C.R. (1975). Molecular biology of amoebic encystment. Indian Journal of Medical Research, 63, 757-767.

Krupp, I. (1966). Immunoelectrophoretic analysis of several strains of *Entamoeba histolytica*. American Journal of Tropical Medicine and Hygiene, 15, 849-854.

Krupp, I.M. (1974a). Comparison of counterimmunoelectrophoresis with other serologic tests in the diagnosis of amebiasis. American Journal of Tropical Medicine and Hygiene, 23, 27-30.

Krupp, I.M. (1974b). Protective immunity to amebic infection demonstrated in guinea pigs. American Journal of Tropical Medicine and Hygiene, 23, 355-360.

Krupp, I.M. (1977). Definition of the antigenic pattern of *Entamoeba histolytica*, and immunoelectrophoretic analysis of the variations of patient response to amebic disease. American Journal of Tropical Medicine and Hygiene, 26, 387-392.

Krupp, I.M. and Powell, J. (1971). Comparative study of the antibody response in amebiasis. American Journal of Tropical Medicine and Hygiene, 20, 421-432.

Kudo, R.R. (1966). Protozoology, 5th edition. Charles C. Thomas, Springfield.

Kuenen, W.A. and Swellengrebel, N.H. (1913). Die Entamöben des Menschen und ihre praktische Bedeutung. Centralblatt für Bakteriologie, 71, 378.

Kusamrarn, T., Sobhon, P. and Bailey, G. (1975a). The mechanism of inhibition-induced ribosome helices in *Entamoeba invadens*. Journal of Cell Biology, 65, 529-539.

Kusamrarn, T., Vinijchaikul, K. and Bailey, G.B. (1975b). Comparison of the structure and function of polysomal and helical ribosomes from *Entamoeba invadens*. Journal of Cell Biology, 65, 540-458.

Lake, J.A. and Slayter, H.S. (1972). Three-dimensional structure of the chromatoid body helix of *Entamoeba invadens*. Journal of Molecular Biology, 66, 271-282.

Landa, L., Capín, R. and Guerrero, M. (1976). Studies on cellular immunity in invasive amebiasis. *In* Proceedings of the International Conference on Amebiasis, Ed. B. Sepúlveda and L.S. Diamond, pp. 661-667. Instituto Mexicano del Seguro Social, Mexico City.

Lee, E., Palacios, O. and Kretschmer, R. (1970). Localización del anticuerpo antiamibiano en las inmunoglobulinas de suero humano. Archivos de Investigación Médica (Mexico), 1, Suppl. s101-s106.

Lesh (Lösch), F.D. (1875). Massive development of amebas in large intestine. Translated and reprinted in American Journal of Tropical Medicine and Hygiene, 24, 383-392, 1975.

Lo, H.S. and Reeves, R.E. (1978). Pyruvate-to-ethanol pathway in *Entamoeba histolytica*. Biochemical Journal, 171, 225-230.

Lo, H.S. and Reeves, R.E. (1979). *Entamoeba histolytica*: Flavins in axenic organisms. Experimental Parasitology, 47, 180-184.

López-Revilla, R. and Gómez, R. (1978). *Entamoeba histolytica, E. invadens*, and *E. moshkovskii*: Fluctuations of the DNA content of axenic trophozoites. Experimental Parasitology, 44, 243-248.

López-Revilla, R. and Saíd-Fernández, S. (1980). Cytopathogenicity of *Entamoeba histolytica*: Hemolytic activity of trophozoite homogenates. American Journal of Tropical Medicine and Hygiene, 29, 209-212.

Lowe, C.Y. and Maegraith, B.G. (1970a). Electron microscopy of *Entamoeba histolytica* in culture. Annals of Tropical Medicine and Parasitology, 64, 283-291.

Lowe, C.Y. and Maegraith, B.G. (1970b). Electron microscopy of an axenic strain of *Entamoeba histolytica*. Annals of Tropical Medicine and Parasitology, 64, 293-298.

Lowe, C.Y. and Maegraith, B.G. (1970c). Electron microscopy of *Entamoeba histolytica* in host tissue. Annals of Tropical Medicine and Parasitology, 64, 469-473.

Ludvík, J. and Shipstone, A.C. (1970). The ultrastructure of *Entamoeba histolytica*. Bulletin of the World Health Organization, 43, 301-308.

Lunde, M.N. and Diamond, L.S. (1969). Studies on antigens from axenically cultivated *Entamoeba histolytica* and *Entamoeba histolytica*-like amebae. American Journal of Tropical Medicine and Hygiene, 18, 1-6.

Lushbaugh, W.B. and Miller, J.H. (1974). Fine structural topochemistry of *Entamoeba histolytica* Schaudinn, 1903. Journal of Parasitology, 60, 421-433.

Lushbaugh, W.B. and Pittman, F.E. (1979). Microscopic observations on the filopodia of *Entamoeba histolytica*. Journal of Protozoology, 26, 186-195.

Lushbaugh, W.B., Kairalla, A.B., Pittman, J.C., Hofbauer, A.F. and Pittman, F.E. (1976). Studies on amebiasis. V. Ultrastructural study of ingestive and digestive processes in *Entamoeba histolytica*: Correlation of freeze-etch replicas and thin sections with enzyme histochemistry. *In* Proceedings of the International Conference on Amebiasis, Ed. B. Sepúlveda and L.S. Diamond, pp. 250-260. Instituto Mexicano del Seguro Social, Mexico City.

Lushbaugh, W.B., Kairalla, A.B., Loadholt, C.B. and Pittman, F.E. (1978). Effect of hamster liver passage on the virulence of axenically cultivated *Entamoeba histolytica*. American Journal of Tropical Medicine and Hygiene, 27, 248-254.

Lushbaugh, W.B., Kairalla, A.B., Cantey, J.R., Hofbauer, A.F. and Pittman, F.E. (1979). Isolation of a cytotoxin-enterotoxin from *Entamoeba histolytica*. Journal of Infectious Diseases, 139, 9-17.

Lushbaugh, W.B., Kairalla, A.B., Hofbauer, A.F., Cantey, J.R. and Pittman, F.E. (1980a). Further studies on a cytotoxin/enterotoxin from *Entamoeba histolytica*. Archivos de Investigación Médica (Mexico), 11, Suppl. 1, 129-133.

Lushbaugh, W.B., Kairalla, A.B., Hofbauer, A.F. and Pittman, F.E. (1980b). Sequential histopathology of cavitary liver abscess formation induced by axenically grown *Entamoeba histolytica*. Archivos de Investigación Médica (Mexico), 11, Suppl. 1, 163-168.

Lushbaugh, W., Kairalla, A.B., Hofbauer, A.F., Arnaud, P., Cantey, J.R. and Pittman, F.E. (1981). Inhibition of *Entamoeba histolytica* cytotoxin by alpha 1 antiprotease and alpha 2 macroglobulins. American Journal of Tropical Medicine and Hygiene, 30, 575-585.

Maddison, S.E., Kagan, I.G. and Elsdon Dew, R. (1968). Comparison of intradermal and serologic tests for the diagnosis of amebiasis. American Journal of Tropical Medicine and Hygiene, 17, 540-547.

Mahajan, R.C. and Ganguly, N.K. (1980). Amoebic antigen in immunodiagnosis and prognosis of amoebic liver abscess. Transactions of the Royal Society of Tropical Medicine and Hygiene, 74, 300-302.

Martínez-Palomo, A. (1978). Inducción de inmunidad protectora antiamibiana con "nuevos" antígenos en el hamster lactante. D. Histopatología. Archivos de Investigación Médica (Mexico), 9, Suppl. 1, 321-324.

Martínez-Palomo, A., González-Robles, A. and de la Torre, M. (1973). Selective agglutination of pathogenic strains of *Entamoeba histolytica* induced by concanavalin A. Nature New Biology, 245, 186-187.

Martínez-Palomo, A., González-Robles, A., de la Torre, M. and de la Hoz, R. (1974). Fijación e inclusión in situ de *E. histolytica*: Aplicaciones en estudios de morfología y citoquímica ultramicroscópica. Archivos de Investigación Médica (Mexico), 5, Suppl. 2, 283-292.

Martínez-Palomo, A., Pinto da Silva, P. and Chávez, B. (1976a). Membrane structure of *Entamoeba histolytica*: Fine structure of freeze-fractured membranes. Journal of Ultrastructural

Research, 54, 148-158.

Martínez-Palomo, A., González-Robles, A. and Chávez de Ramírez, B. (1976b). Ultrastructural study of various *Entamoeba* strains. *In* Proceedings of the International Conference on Amebiasis, Ed. B. Sepúlveda and L.S. Diamond, pp. 226-237. Instituto Mexicano del Seguro Social, Mexico City.

Martínez-Palomo, A., Meza, I., Beaty, G. and Cereijido, M. (1980a). Experimental modulation of occluding junctions in a cultured transporting epithelium. Journal of Cell Biology, 87, 736-745.

Martínez-Palomo, A., Orozco, E. and González-Robles, A. (1980b). *Entamoeba histolytica*: Topochemistry and dynamics of the cell surface. *In* The Host-Invader Interplay, Ed. H. Van den Bossche, pp. 55-68. Elsevier/North Holland Biomedical Press, Amsterdam.

Martínez-Palomo, A., Tanimoto-Weki, M. and Tena-Betancourt, B.E. (1980c). Evolución de las lesiones producidas en hámsters por inoculación de *Entamoeba histolytica*. Archivos de Investigación Médica (Mexico), 11, Suppl. 1, 169-172.

Mathis, C. and Mercier, L. (1916). La division simple chez *Entamoeba dysenteriae*. Comptes Rendus des Séances de la Société de Biologie (Paris), 79, 982-984.

Mattern, C.F.T. and Keister, D.B. (1977). Experimental amebiasis. II. Hepatic amebiasis in the newborn hamster. American Journal of Tropical Medicine and Hygiene, 26, 402-411.

Mattern, C.F.T., Diamond, L.S. and Daniel, W.A. (1972). Viruses of *Entamoeba histolytica*. II. Morphogenesis of the polyhedral particle $(ABRM_2 \rightarrow HK-9) \rightarrow HB-301$ and the filamentous agent $(ABRM)_2 \rightarrow HK-9$. Journal of Virology, 9, 342-358.

Mattern, C.F.T., Diamond, L.S., Daniel, W.A. and Keister, D.B. (1976). Unusual variation of "normal" cytoplasmic bars of *Entamoeba histolytica*. *In* Proceedings of the International Conference on Amebiasis, Ed. B. Sepúlveda and L.S. Diamond, pp. 346-357. Instituto Mexicano del Seguro Social, Mexico City.

Mattern, C.F.T., Keister, D.B. and Diamond, L.S. (1979). Experimental amebiasis. IV. Amebal viruses and the virulence of *Entamoeba histolytica*. American Journal of Tropical Medicine and

Hygiene, 28, 653-657.

Mattern, C.F.T., Keister, D.B. and Caspar Natovitz, P. (1980). *Entamoeba histolytica* "toxin": Fetuin neutralizable and lectin-like. American Journal of Tropical Medicine and Hygiene, 29, 26-30.

McCaul, T.F. (1977). Transmission electron microscopy observations of phagocytosis in trophozoites of *Entamoeba histolytica* in contact with tissue culture cells. Zeitschrift für Parasitenkunde, 52, 203-211.

McCaul, T.F. and Bird, R.G. (1977). Surface features of *Entamoeba histolytica* and rabbit kidney (RK13) cell surface changes after trophozoite contact-observations by scanning electron microscopy. International Journal for Parasitology, 7, 383-388.

McCaul, T.F., Poston, R.N. and Bird, R.G. (1977). *Entamoeba histolytica* and *Entamoeba invadens*: Chromium release from labeled human liver cells in culture. Experimental Parasitology, 43, 342-352.

McConnachie, E.W. (1969). The morphology, formation and development of cysts of *Entamoeba*. Parasitology, 59, 41-53.

McLaughlin, J. and Meerovitch, E. (1975a). The surface and cytoplasmic membranes of *Entamoeba invadens* (Rodhain 1934). I. Gross chemical and enzymatic properties. Comparative Biochemistry and Physiology, 52B, 477-486.

McLaughlin, J. and Meerovitch, E. (1975b). The surface and cytoplasmic membranes of *Entamoeba invadens* (Rodhain 1934). II. Polypeptide and phospholipid composition. Comparative Biochemistry and Physiology, 52B, 487-497.

Meerovitch, E. and Ghadirian, E. (1978). Restoration of virulence of axenically cultivated *Entamoeba histolytica* by cholesterol. Canadian Journal of Microbiology, 24, 63-65.

Meerovitch, E., Hartman, D.P. and Ghadirian, E. (1978). Protective immunity and possible autoimmune regulation in amebiasis. Archivos de Investigación Médica (Mexico), 9, Suppl. 1, 247-252.

Michel, R. and Hohmann, R. (1979). Der Einfluss von Cytochalasin B. Colchicin und Vinblastin auf die Adhäsion von *Entamoeba histolytica*. Zeitschrift für Parasitenkunde, 60, 123-133.

Michel, R. and Schupp, E. (1975). Fibrilläre and Tubuläre Feinstrukturen im Cytoplasma von *Entamoeba histolytica*. Zeitschrift für Parasitenkunde, 47, 11-21.

Miller, J.H. and Deas, J.E. (1971). Observations on the cysts of *Entamoeba histolytica*. Proceedings of the Annual Electron Microscopic Society of America Meeting, 28, 124-125.

Miller, J.H., Swartzwelder, J.C. and Deas, J.E. (1961). An electron microscopic study of *Entamoeba histolytica*. Journal of Parasitology, 47, 577-579.

Miller, M.J., Scott, F. and Foster, E.F. (1973). An evaluation of immunological indicators for amebic disease prevalence. American Journal of Tropical Medicine and Hygiene, 22, 331-336.

Montalvo, F.E., Reeves, R.E. and Warren, L.G. (1971). Aerobic and anaerobic metabolism in *Entamoeba histolytica*. Experimental Parasitology, 30, 249-256.

Mora Galindo, J., Martínez-Palomo, A. and Chávez, B. (1978). Interacción entre *Entamoeba histolytica* y el epitelio cecal del cobayo. Archivos de Investigación Médica (Mexico), 9, Suppl. 1, 261-274.

Morgan, R.S., Slayter, H.S. and Weller, D.L. (1968). Isolation of ribosomes from cysts of *Entamoeba invadens*. Journal of Cell Biology, 36, 45-51.

Muñoz, M.L., Calderón, J. and Rojkind, M. (1982). The collagenase of *Entamoeba histolytica*. Journal of Experimental Medicine. In Press.

Narasimhamurti, C.C. (1964). Nuclear division in *Entamoeba invadens* Rodhain, 1934. Parasitology, 54, 95-103.

Neal, R.A. (1957). Virulence of *Entamoeba histolytica*. Transactions of the Royal Society of Tropical Medicine and Hygiene, 51, 313-319.

Neal, R.A. (1966). Experimental studies on *Entamoeba* with special reference to speciation. Advances in Parasitology, 4, 1-51.

Orozco, E., Martínez-Palomo, A. and López-Revilla, R. (1978). Un modelo in vitro para el estudio cuantitativo de la virulencia de *Entamoeba histolytica*. Archivos de Investigación Médica (Mexico), 9, Suppl. 1, 257-260.

Orozco Orozco, M.E., Martínez-Palomo, A. and Guarneros, G. (1980). Virulencia y propiedades de superficie de varias cepas axénicas de *Entamoeba histolytica*. Archivos de Investigación Médica (Mexico), 11, Suppl. 1, 153-158.

Ortiz-Ortiz, L., Garmilla, C., Tanimoto-Weki, M. and Zamacona, R. G. (1973). Hipersensibilidad celular en amibiasis. I. Reacciones en hámsters inoculados con *E. histolytica*. Archivos de Investigación Médica (Mexico), 4, Suppl. 1, 141-146.

Ortiz-Ortiz, L., Gómez, R. and Estrada-Parra, S. (1974). ¿Existen complejos inmunes en el suero de pacientes con absceso hepático amibiano? Archivos de Investigación Médica (Mexico), 5, Suppl. 2, 491-500.

Ortiz-Ortiz, L., Zamacona, G., Sepúlveda, B. and Capín, R.N. (1975). Cell-mediated immunity in patients with amebic abscess of the liver. Clinical Immunology and Immunopathology, 4, 127-134.

Ortiz-Ortiz, L., Capín, R., Capín, N.R., Sepúlveda, B. and Zamacona, G. (1978). Activation of the alternative pathway of complement by *Entamoeba histolytica*. Clinical and Experimental Immunology, 34, 10-18.

Osada, M. (1959). Electron-microscopic studies on protozoa. I. Fine structure of *Entamoeba histolytica*. Keio Journal of Medicine, 8, 99-108.

O'Shea, M.S. and Feria-Velasco, A. (1974). Demostración ultramicroscópica de antígenos de superficie en trofozoítos de *E. histolytica* por inmunofluorescencias con IgG humana específica. Archivos de Investigación Médica (Mexico), 5, Suppl. 2, 307-314.

Palacios, O., de la Hoz, R. and Sosa, H. (1978). Determinación del antígeno amibiano en heces por el método ELISA (enzyme linked immunosorbent assay) para la identificación de *Entamoeba histolytica*. Archivos de Investigación Médica (Mexico), 9, Suppl. 1, 339-348.

Pan, C.T. and Geiman, G.M. (1955). Comparative studies of intestinal amebae. I. Distributions and cyclic changes of the nucleic acids in *Endamoeba histolytica* and *Endamoeba coli*. American Journal of Hygiene, 62, 66-79.

Perches, A., Kretschmer, R., Lee, E. and Sepúlveda, B. (1970). Determinación de inmunoglobulinas del suero en pacientes con amibiasis invasora. Archivos de Investigación Médica (Mexico), 1, Suppl., s97-s100.

Phillips, B.P., Diamond, L.S., Bartgis, I.L. and Stuppler, S.A. (1972). Results of intracecal inoculation of germfree and conventional guinea pigs and germfree rats with axenically cultivated *Entamoeba histolytica*. Journal of Protozoology, 19, 498-499.

Pigon, A. (1978). Origin of medium exudate and its effect on cell surface in *Acanthamoeba* culture. Cytobiologie, 16, 259-267.

Pinto da Silva, P. and Martínez-Palomo, A. (1974). Induced redistribution of membrane particles, anionic sites and con A receptors in *Entamoeba histolytica*. Nature, 249, 170-171.

Pinto da Silva, P., Martínez-Palomo, A. and González-Robles, A. (1975). Membrane structure and surface coat of *Entamoeba histolytica*. Topochemistry and dynamics of the cell surface: Cap formation and microexudate. Journal of Cell Biology, 64, 538-550.

Pollard, T.D. and Maupin, P. (1978). Electron microscopy of contractile proteins. In Electron Microscopy 1978, Ed. J.M. Sturgess, 3, 606-614. Microscopical Society of Canada, Toronto.

Prathap, K. and Gilman, R. (1970). The histopathology of acute intestinal amebiasis. American Journal of Pathology, 60, 229-246.

Proctor, E.M. (1976). Ultrastructure of trophozoites of *Entamoeba histolytica* from human amoebic liver abscess. Transactions of the Royal Society of Tropical Medicine and Hygiene, 70, 256-257.

Proctor, E.M. and Gregory, M.A. (1972). The observation of a surface active lysosome in the trophozoites of *Entamoeba histolytica* from the human colon. Annals of Tropical Medicine and Parasitology, 66, 339-342.

Proctor, E.M. and Gregory, M.A. (1973). The surface active lysosome of *Entamoeba histolytica*. International Journal of Parasitology, 3, 274-

Rajaraman, R., Raunds, D.E., Ye, S.P.S. and Rembaum, A. (1974). A scanning electron microscope study of cell adhesion and spreading in vitro. Experimental Cell Research, 88, 327-339.

Ravdin, J.I., Croft, B.Y. and Guerrant, R.L. (1980). Cytopathogenic mechanisms of *Entamoeba histolytica*. Journal of Experimental Medicine, 152, 377-390.

Reeves, R.E. and Bischoff, J.M. (1968). Classification of *Entamoeba* species by means of electrophoretic properties of amebal enzymes. Journal of Parasitology, 54, 594-600.

Reeves, R.E. and West, B. (1980). *Entamoeba histolytica*: Nucleic acid precursors affecting axenic growth. Experimental Parasitology, 49, 78-82.

Reeves, R.E., Lushbaugh, T.S. and Montalvo, F.F. (1971). Characterization of deoxyribonucleic acid of *Entamoeba histolytica* by cesium chloride density centrifugation. Journal of Parasitology, 57, 939-944.

Rengpien, S. and Bailey, G.B. (1975). Differentiation of *Entamoeba*: A new medium and optimal conditions for axenic encystation of *E. invadens*. Journal of Parasitology, 61, 24-30.

Richards, C.S., Goldman, M. and Cannon, L.T. (1966). Cultivation of *Entamoeba histolytica* and *Entamoeba histolytica*-like strains at reduced temperature and behaviour of the amebae in diluted media. American Journal of Tropical Medicine and Hygiene, 15, 648-655.

Robinson, G.L. (1968). The laboratory diagnosis of human parasitic amoebae. Transactions of the Royal Society of Tropical Medicine and Hygiene, 62, 285-294.

Rondanelli, E.G., Osculati, F., Gerna, G. and Fiori, G.P. (1965). Ricerche microelettroniche su *Entamoeba invadens*. Bolletino dell'Istituto Sieroterapico Milanese, 44, 218-239.

Rondanelli, E.G., Osculati, F. and Gerna, G. (1966). Aspetti ultrastrutturali di *Entamoeba histolytica*. Ricerche microelettroniche. Bollettino dell'Istituto Sieroterapico Milanese, 45, 279-290.

Rondanelli, E.G., Carosi, G., Filice, G. and de Carneri, I. (1974). Observations of surface active lysosomes and other organelles in monoxenically cultivated trophozoites of *Entamoeba histolytica* and *Entamoeba coli*. International Journal for Parasitology, 4, 433-435.

Rondanelli, E.G., Carosi, G., Filice, C., Carnevale, G., Scaglia, M. and Barbarini, G. (1977). Ultrastruttura di *Entamoeba histolytica*. Giarnale di Malattie Infettive e Parassitarie, 29, 592-606.

Rosas, G.A. and Najarian, H.H. (1965). Infectivity studies on the Laredo strain of *Entamoeba histolytica*. Texas Reports on Biology and Medicine, 23, 507-511.

Rosenbaum, R.M. and Wittner, M. (1970). Ultrastructure of bacterized and axenic trophozoites of *Entamoeba histolytica* with particular reference to helical bodies. Journal of Cell Biology, 45, 367-382.

Ruiz Castañeda, M., de la Torre, M. and Aubanel, M. (1976). Investigación de antígeno circulante en amibiasis invasora. Gaceta Médica de México, 112, 393-396.

Saíd Fernández, S. and López-Revilla, R. (1978). Characteristic protein electrophoretic patterns of four *Entamoeba* strains. Zeitschrift für Parasitenkunde, 56, 219-225.

Sanderson, C.J. (1976). The mechanism of T cell mediated cytotoxicity. II. Morphological studies of cell death by time-lapse microcinematography. Proceedings of the Royal Society of London. Series B, 192, 241-255.

Sargeaunt, P.G. and Williams, J.E. (1978). Electrophoretic isoenzyme patterns of *Entamoeba histolytica* and *Entamoeba coli*. Transactions of the Royal Society of Tropical Medicine and Hygiene, 72, 164-166.

Sargeaunt, P.G. and Williams, J.E. (1979). Electrophoretic isoenzyme patterns of the pathogenic and non-pathogenic intestinal amoebae of man. Transactions of the Royal Society of Tropical Medicine and Hygiene, 73, 225-227.

Sargeaunt, P.G., Williams, J.E. and Grene, J.D. (1978). The differentiation of invasive and non-invasive *Entamoeba histolytica* by isoenzyme electrophoresis. Transactions of the Royal Society of Tropical Medicine and Hygiene, 72, 519-521.

Sargeaunt, P.G., Williams, J.E. and Neal, R.A. (1980a). A comparative study of *Entamoeba histolytica* (NIH:200, HK9, etc.), "*E. histolytica*-like" and other morphologically identical amoebae using isoenzyme electrophoresis. Transactions of the Royal Society of Tropical Medicine and Hygiene, 74, 469-474.

Sargeaunt, P.G., Williams, J.E., Kumate, J. and Jimenez, E. (1980b). The epidemiology of *Entamoeba histolytica* in Mexico City. A pilot survey I. Transactions of the Royal Society of Tropical Medicine and Hygiene, 74, 653-656.

Savanat, T., Bunnag, D., Chongsuphajaisiddhi, T. and Viriyanond, P. (1973a). Skin test for amebiasis: An appraisal. American Journal of Tropical Medicine and Hygiene, 22, 168-173.

Savanat, T., Viriyanond, P. and Nimitmongkol, N. (1973b). Blast transformation of lymphocytes in amebiasis. American Journal of Tropical Medicine and Hygiene, 22, 705-710.

Sawhney, S., Chakravarti, R.N., Jain, P. and Vinayak, V.K. (1980). Immunogenicity of axenic *Entamoeba histolytica* antigen and its fractions. Transactions of the Royal Society of Tropical Medicine and Hygiene, 74, 26-29.

Sawyer, M.K., Bischoff, J.M., Guidry, M.A. and Reeves, R.E. (1967). Lipids from *Entamoeba histolytica*. Experimental Parasitology, 20, 295-302.

Schaudinn, F. (1903). Untersuchungen über die Fortpflanzung eininger Rhizopoden. Arbeiten aus dem Kaiserlichen Gesundeitsamte, 19, 547-576.

Schmuñis, G.A., Szarfman, A., De Souza, W. and Langembach, T. (1980). *Trypanosoma cruzi*: Antibody-induced mobility of surface antigens. Experimental Parasitology, 50, 90-102.

Segovia, E., Capin, R. and Landa, L. (1980). Transformación blastoide de linfocitos estimulados con antígeno lisosomal en pacientes con amibiasis intestinal. Archivos de Investigación Médica (Mexico), 11, Suppl. 1, 225-228.

Sen, A., Ghosh, S.N., Mukerjee, S. and Ray, J.C. (1961). Antigenic structure of *Entamoeba histolytica*. Nature, 192, 893.

Sepúlveda, B. (1970). Reacciones de hemaglutinación y de precipitación con antígeno amibiano axenico en amibiasis invasora. Archivos de Investigación Médica (Mexico), 1, Suppl., s111-s116.

Sepúlveda, B. (1976). Immunology of amebiasis. *In* Proceedings of the International Conference on Amebiasis, Ed. B. Sepúlveda and L.S. Diamond, pp. 686-702. Instituto Mexicano del Seguro Social, Mexico City.

Sepúlveda, B. and Martínez-Palomo, A. (1982). The immunology of amoebiasis produced by *Entamocba histolytica*. *In* Immunology of Parasitic Infections, Ed. S. Cohen and K.S. Warren. Blackwell Scientific Publications, Oxford. In press.

Sepúlveda, B., Lee, E., de la Torre, M. and Landa, L. (1971). El diagnóstico serológico de la amibiasis invasora con la técnica de la inmunoelectroforesis cruzada. Archivos de Investigación Médica (Mexico), 2, Suppl., 263-268.

Sepúlveda, B., Aubanel, M., Landa, L. and Velázquez, G. (1972). Avances en la técnica de contra-inmunoelectroforesis para el estudio serológico de la amibiasis. Archivos de Investigación Médica (Mexico), 3, Suppl. 2, 363-370.

Sepúlveda, B., Chévez, A., Iturbe-Alessio, I. and Ortiz-Ortiz, L. (1973a). Efecto de la gammaglobulina inmune antiamibiana sobre el trofozoíto de *E. histolytica*. Archivos de Investigación Médica (Mexico), 4, Suppl., 1, s79-s86.

Sepúlveda, B., Tanimoto-Weki, M., Guerrero, A. and Solís, G. (1973b). Inmunidad en hamsters consecutiva a vacunación con cultivos monoxénicos y axénicos de *E. histolytica*. Archivos de Investigación Médica (Mexico), 4, Suppl. 1, s159-s164.

Sepúlveda, B., Ortiz-Ortiz, L., Chévez, A. and Segura, M. (1974a). Comprobación de la naturaleza inmunológica del efecto del suero y de la gammaglobulina inmunes sobre el trofozoíto de *E. histolytica*. Archivos de Investigación Médica (Mexico), 5, Suppl. 2, 343-346.

Sepúlveda, B., Tanimoto-Weki, M., Calderón, P. and de la Hoz, R. (1974b). Inducción de inmunidad pasiva antiamibiana en el hamster por la inyección de suero inmune. Archivos de Investigación Médica (Mexico), 5, Suppl. 2, 451-456.

Sepúlveda, B., Arroyo-Begovich, A., Tanimoto-Weki, M., Martínez-Palomo, A. and Ortiz-Ortiz, L. (1978). Inducción de inmunidad protectora antiamibiana con "nuevos" antígenos en el hamster lactante. Archivos de Investigación Médica (Mexico), 9, Suppl. 1, 309-328.

Serrano, R. and Reeves, R.E. (1974). Glucose transport in *Entamoeba histolytica*. Biochemical Journal, 144, 43-48.

Serrano, R. and Reeves, R.E. (1975). Physiological significance of glucose transport in *Entamoeba histolytica*. Experimental Parasitology, 37, 411-416.

Serrano, R., Deas, J.E. and Warren, L.G. (1977). *Entamoeba histolytica*: Membrane fractions. Experimental Parasitology, 41, 370-384.

Sharma, R. (1959). Effect of cholesterol on growth and virulence of *E. histolytica*. Transactions of the Royal Society of Tropical Medicine and Hygiene, 53, 278-281.

Sharma, S.D. and Piessens, W.F. (1978). Tumor cell killing by macrophages activated in vitro with lymphocyte mediators. III. Inhibition by cytochalasins, colchicine, and vinblastine. Cellular Immunology, 38, 276-285.

Sharma, N.N., Albach, R.A. and Schaffer, J.G. (1970). Cytochemical comparison of nucleoproteins and acid mucopolysaccharide in axenic vs. monoxenic *Entamoeba histolytica*. Bacteriological Proceedings, 20.

Siddiqui, W.A. and Rudzinska, M.A. (1965). The fine structure of axenically grown trophozoites of *Entamoeba invadens* with special reference to the nucleus and helical ribonucleoprotein bodies. Journal of Protozoology, 12, 448-459.

Singh, B.N. (1952). Nuclear division in nine species of small free-living amoebae and its bearing on the classification of the order *Amoebida*. Philosophical Transactions of the Royal Society. Series B, 236, 405-461.

Snyder, T.L. and Meleney, H.E. (1946). Migration of *Entamoeba histolytica* on solid media. Journal of Parasitology, 32, 354-358.

Sobota, A., Przelecka, A. and Janossy, A.G.S. (1978). X-ray microanalysis of calcium-dependent deposits at the plasma membrane of *Acanthamoeba castellanii*. Cytobiologie, 17, 464-469.

Spencer, F.M. and Monroe, L.S. (1961). Color Atlas of Intestinal Parasites, pp. 22-28. Charles C. Thomas, Springfield.

Swartzwelder, J.C. and Avant, W.H. (1952). Immunity to amebic infection in dogs. American Journal of Tropical Medicine and Hygiene, 1, 567-575.

Swellengrebel, N.H. (1961). L'écologie d'*Entamoeba histolytica* et l'épidemiologie de l'amibiase. Bulletin de la Société de Pathologie Exotique, 54, 459-466.

Takeuchi, T., Weinbach, E.C. and Diamond, L.S. (1977). *Entamoeba histolytica*: Localization and characterization of phosphoglucomutase, uridine diphosphate glucose pyrophosphorylase, and glycogen synthase. Experimental Parasitology, 43, 115-121.

Tanabe, M. (1934). The excystation and metacystic development of *Entamoeba histolytica* in the intestine of white rats. Keijo Journal of Medicine, 5, 238-253.

Tanimoto, M., Sepúlveda, B., Vázquez-Saavedra, J.A. and Landa, L. (1971). Lesiones producidas en el hígado del hamster por inoculación de *Entamoeba histolytica* cultivada en medio axénico. Archivos de Investigación Médica (Mexico), 2, Suppl. 1, 275-284.

Tanimoto-Weki, M., Vázquez-Saavedra, J., Calderón, P. and Aguirre-García, J. (1973). Inmunidad consecutiva a la inyección de antígeno amibiano axénico en el hamster. Archivos de Investigación Médica (Mexico), 4, Suppl. 1, s147-s154.

Tanimoto-Weki, M., Calderón, P., de la Hoz, R. and Aguirre-García, J. (1974). Inoculación de trofozoítos de *E. histolytica* en hamster bajo la acción de drogas inmunosupresoras. Archivos de Investigación Médica (Mexico), 5, Suppl. 2, 441-446.

Tanowitz, H.B., Wittner, M., Rosenbaum, R.M. and Kress, Y. (1975). In vitro studies on the differential toxicity of metronidazole in protozoa and mammalian cells. Annals of Tropical Medicine and Parasitology, 69, 19-28.

Thepsuparungskikul, V., Seng, L. and Bailey, G.B. (1971). Differentiation of *Entamoeba*: Encystation of *E. invadens* in monoxenic and axenic cultures. Journal of Parasitology, 57, 1288-1291.

Treviño-García Manzo, N., de la Torre, M., Ruiz de Chávez, I., Hernández-López, H. and Escobedo, A. (1970). Morfología de *Entamoeba histolytica* en el absceso hepático del hamster. Archivos de Investigación Médica (Mexico), 1, Suppl., 61-80.

Treviño-García Manzo, N., Feria-Velasco, A., Ruiz de Chávez, I. and de la Torre, M. (1971). Lisosomas en *Entamoeba histolytica*. Archivos de Investigación Médica (Mexico), 2, Suppl., 179-186.

Trissl, D., Martínez-Palomo, A. and Chávez, B. (1976). Isolation of intact *Entamoeba* surface coat and caps induced by concanavalin A. Journal of Cell Biology, 70, 417a.

Trissl, D., Martínez-Palomo, A., Argüello, C., de la Torre, M. and de la Hoz, R. (1977). Surface properties related to concanavalin A-induced agglutination. A comparative study of several *Entamoeba* strains. Journal of Experimental Medicine, 145, 652-665.

Trissl, D., Martínez-Palomo, A., de la Torre, M., de la Hoz, R. and Pérez de Suárez, E. (1978). Surface properties of *Entamoeba*: Increased rates of human erythrocyte phagocytosis in pathogenic strains. Journal of Experimental Medicine, 148, 1137-1145.

Uribe, C. (1926). Nuclear division in the trophozoites of *Endamoeba histolytica*. Proceedings of the National Academy of Sciences, 12, 305-311.

Van Steenis, P.B. (1957). The problem of the minuta forms in amoebic dysentery and amoebiasis. Documenta de Medicina Geographica et Tropica, 9, 325-330.

Van Thiel, P.H. (1961). Reconciliation entre les conceptions concernant la biologie de l'*Entamoeba histolytica* en rapport avec la perturbation de l'équilibre entre l'homme et le parasite par le traitement médical. Bulletin de la Société de Pathologie Exotique, 54, 824-829.

Vázquez-Saavedra, J., Tanimoto-Weki, M., Olivera-López, J.I., Caracheo-Reyes, F. and Cortés-Arcos, A. (1973). Inmunidad consecutiva a infección amibiana curada en el hamster. Archivos de Investigación Médica (Mexico), 4, Suppl. 1, s155-s158.

Villarejos, V.M. (1962). Studies on the pathogenicity of *Entamoeba histolytica* and other ameba species. Tropical Diseases Bulletin, 59, 780-781.

Vinayak, V.K. and Chitkara, N.L. (1976). Selective ability of *Entamoeba histolytica* to haemolyse red blood cells. A preliminary communication. Indian Journal of Medical Research, 64, 1443-1445.

Vinayak, V.K., Sawhney, S., Jain, P. and Chakravarti, R.N. (1980). Protective effects of crude and chromatographic fractions of axenic *Entamoeba histolytica* in guinea-pigs. Transactions of the Royal Society of Tropical Medicine and Hygiene, 74, 483-487.

Wagner, R.R. (1975). Reproduction of rhabdoviruses. *In* Comprehensive Virology, Ed. H. Fraenkel-Conrat and R.R. Wagner, pp. 1-94. Plenum Press, New York.

Walker, E.L. and Sellards, A.W. (1913). Experimental entamoebic dysentery. Philippine Journal of Science. B, Tropical Medicine, 8, 253-330.

Weinbach, E.C. and Diamond, L.S. (1974). *Entamoeba histolytica*: I. Aerobic metabolism. Experimental Parasitology, 35, 232-243.

Weinbach, E.C., Harlow, D.R., Takeuchi, T., Diamond, L.S., Claggett, C.E. and Kon, H. (1976). Aerobic metabolism of *Entamoeba histolytica*: Facts and fallacies. In Proceedings of the International Conference on Amebiasis, Ed. B. Sepúlveda and L.S. Diamond, pp. 190-203. Instituto Mexicano del Seguro Social, Mexico City.

Weinbach, E.C., Harlow, D.R., Claggett, C.E. and Diamond, L.S. (1977). *Entamoeba histolytica*: Diaphorase activities. Experimental Parasitology, 41, 186-197.

Westphal, A. and Michel, R. (1971). Phagozytose und Pinozytose der *Entamoeba histolytica*. Zeitschrift für Tropenmedizin und Parasitologie, 22, 82-91.

Wijesundera, M. de S. (1980). Hepatic amoebiasis in immunodepressed mice. Transactions of the Royal Society of Tropical Medicine and Hygiene, 74, 216-220.

Wittner, M. (1968). Growth characteristics of axenic strains of *Entamoeba histolytica*, Schaudinn, 1903. Journal of Protozoology, 15, 403-406.

Wittner, M. and Rosenbaum, R.M. (1970). Role of bacteria in modifying virulence of *Entamoeba histolytica*. Studies of amebae from axenic cultures. American Journal of Tropical Medicine and Hygiene, 19, 755-761.

Wood, H.G. (1977). Some reactions in which inorganic pyrophosphate replaces ATP and serves as a source of energy. Federation Proceedings, 36, 2197-2205.

World Health Organization. (1969). Amoebiasis. Report of a WHO Expert Committee. World Health Organization Technical Report Series, No. 421.

Zaman, E. (1961). An electron-microscopic observation of the "tail" end of *Entamoeba invadens*. Transactions of the Royal Society of Tropical Medicine and Hygiene, 55, 263-264.

Zaman, V. (1972). Structure and movement of *Entamoeba*. Annals of Tropical Medicine and Parasitology, 66, 329-333.

Zaman, V. (1973). The intranuclear bodies of *Entamoeba*. International Journal of Parasitology, 3, 243-251.

CHAPTER 9
Selected Monographs and Articles on Amebiasis

9.1 History of Amebiasis

Beltrán, E. (1974). Notas de historia protozoológica. IV. Las amibas parásitas. Anales de la Sociedad Mexicana de Historia de la Ciencia y de la Tecnología. (Mexico), 4, 259-308.

Bloomfield, A.L. (1957). A bibliography of internal medicine: Amebic dysentery. Journal of Chronic Diseases, 5, 235-252.

Dobell, C. (1919). The Amoebae Living in Man. A Zoological Monograph. John Bale, Sons & Danielsson, London.

Fournier Villada, R. (1956). Bibliografía Mexicana del Absceso Hepático. La Prensa Médica Mexicana, Mexico City.

Imperato, P.J. (1981). A historical overview of amebiasis. Bulletin of the New York Academy of Medicine, 57, 175-187.

Kean, B.H., Mott, K.E. and Russell, A.J., Eds. (1978). Amoebiasis. In Tropical Medicine and Parasitology, Classic Investigations, 1, 71-167. Cornell University Press, Ithaca.

Martínez-Báez, M. (1966). The history of amebiasis. In Proceedings of the International Conference on Amebiasis, Ed. B. Sepúlveda and L.S. Diamond, pp. 53-63. Instituto Mexicano del Seguro Social, Mexico City.

Sepúlveda, B. (1976). La contribución de Don Miguel Jiménez al estudio del absceso hepático. Gaceta Médica de México, 112, 259- 262.

Stilwell, G.G. (1955). Amebiasis: Its early history. Gastroenterology, 28, 606-622.

9.2 Clinical Aspects of Amebiasis

Adams, E.B. and MacLeod, I.N. (1977). I. Amebic dysentery and its complications. II. Amebic liver abscess and its complications. Medicine, 56, 315-334.

Anderson, H.H., Bostick, W.L. and Johnstone, H.G. (1953). Amebiasis. Pathology, Diagnosis and Chemotherapy. Charles C. Thomas, Springfield.

Brandt, H. and Pérez-Tamayo, R. (1970). Amibiasis. La Prensa Médica Mexicana Mexico City.

Deschiens, R. (1965). L'Amibiase et L'Amibe Dysentérique. Masson, Paris.

Elsdon-Dew, R. (1968). The epidemiology of amoebiasis. Advances in Parasitology, 6, 1-62.

Guarner, V. (1974). La evolución de los conceptos en el tratamiento quirúrgico de la amibiasis invasora del hígado. Archivos de Investigación Médica (Mexico), 5, Suppl. 2, 549-552.

Juniper, K. (1978). Amoebiasis. Clinics in Gastroenterology, 7, 3-29.

Knight, R. (1979). Amebiasis *In* Cecil Textbook of Medicine, Ed. P.B. Beeson, W. McDermott, and J.B. Wyngaarden, 15 Ed. pp. 589-594. Saunders, Philadelphia.

Krogstad, D.J., Spencer, H.C. and Healy, G.R. (1978). Amebiasis. New England Journal of Medicine, 289, 262-265.

Krogstad, D.J., Spencer, H.C., Healy, G.R., Gleason, N.S., Sexton, D.J. and Herron, C.A. (1978). Amebiasis: Epidemiologic studies in the United States. Annals of Internal Medicine, 88, 89-97.

Mahmoud, A.A.F. and Warren, K.S. (1976). Algorithms in the diagnosis and management of exotic diseases. XVII. Amebiasis. Journal of Infectious Diseases, 134, 639-643.

O'Farril Bautista, J. (1976). Surgical treatment of invasive amebiasis. *In* Proceedings of the International Conference on Amebiasis, Ed. B. Sepúlveda and L.S. Diamond, pp. 888-892. Instituto Mexicano del Seguro Social, Mexico City.

Perches, A., Nieves, M., Landa, L. and Sepúlveda, B. (1976). Chemotherapy of amebic liver abscess. *In* Procedings of the International Conference on Amebiasis. Ed. B. Sepúlveda and L.S. Diamond, pp. 878-880. Instituto Mexicano del Seguro Social, Mexico City.

Pérez-Tamayo, R. and Brandt, H. (1971). Amebiasis. *In* Pathology of Protozoal and Helminthic Diseases, Ed. R.A. Marcial-Rojas, pp. 145-187. Robert E. Krieger, Huntington.

Sepúlveda, B. (1970). La amibiasis invasora por *Entamoeba histolytica*. Gaceta Médica de México, 100, 201-254.

Sepúlveda, B. and Martínez-Palomo, A. (1982). Immunology of amoebiasis produced by *Entamoeba histolytica*. *In* Immunology of Parasitic Infections, Ed. S. Cohen and K.S. Warren. Blackwell, Oxford.

Shaffer, J.G., Shlaes, W.H. and Radke, R.A. (1965). Amebiasis: A Biomedical Problem. Charles C. Thomas, Springfield.

United States Department of Health, Education, and Welfare. (1976). Amebiasis. Laboratory Diagnosis. Public Health Service Publication 1187, Washington. D.C.

Wilmot, A.J. (1962). Clinical Amoebiasis. Blackwell Scientific Publications, London.

Index

Acanthamoeba, 25,40,65
Acid phosphatase, 13,49
Agglutination, 97
Amebiasis,
   clinical classifica-
      tion, 1
   clinical importance, 2
   epidemiology, 2,74,78
   history, 1,2
   immunology, 85-94
   incidence, 2,95
   intestinal, 1, 103-105
   invasive, 1,74,77,82
      89,95
   lumenal, 1,105
   pathology, 120
   unsolved problems, 119
Antibodies, 41,88,89
Antigens,
   characterization, 85, 86,89
   mobility, 41,87
   subcellular location, 32,67,87
Antigen-antibody complexes, 86
Attachment, 44,47,103,104

Bacteria, effect on virulence, 99
   100
Biochemical taxonomy, 81
Biochemistry, 61-71

Capping, 38,90,96,108
Carriers, 55,78,80,83,89
Cell biology, 5-59
Cell division, 55
Cell surface, 32
Cellular immune reaction, 91
Ceramide aminoethyl phos-
   phonate, 65
Cholesterol, and virulence,
   101
Chromatin, 50,51,58
Chromatoid bodies, 19-23,58,
   71
Chromosomes, 50,53
Commensal phase, 1,105
Complement system, 89,90,
   108
Concanavalin A, 32,66,67,91,
   97
Counterimmunoelectropho-
   resis, 88
Cultures, axenic, 68-70,85,96,
   98,100
Culture conditions, and viru-
   lence, 101
Cylindrical bodies, 27-30
Cysteine, 68
Cysts, 20,27,56-59,70,119
Cytoplasm, 11

Cytoskeleton, 25-27
Cytotoxic effect, 27,44,65,109-117

Delayed hypersensitivity, 91
Dense oval bodies, 41
Differentiation, 70,71
DNA, 51,81

ELISA technique, 86
Encystation, 20,56,58,71
Endocytosis, 38,43,47,61
Endoplasmic reticulum, 11,17
Endosome, 50,51
Entamoeba classification, 73
Entamoeba coli, 1,29,41,49,73,82
Entamoeba dispar, 2,77,79,80
Entamoeba dysenteriae, 2,77
Entamoeba hartmanii, 2,5,73,74
Entamoeba histolytica,
  biochemical taxonomy, 77
  carrier strains, 74,80,83
  diameter, 5
  DNA, 81
  erythrophagocytic, 73
  invasive strains, 74,80,83
  life cycle, 56
  locomotion, 8-10
  minuta form, 73
  morphology, 5,8,11
  strain variations, 70,74,76-78,82
E. histolytica-like, Laredo, 26,29, 55,70,74,79,81,82
Entamoeba invadens, 19,20,23,27, 29,41,65,70,81,82
Entamoeba gingivalis, 29,73
Entamoeba moshkovskii, 22,41,49, 55,70,74,79,81,82
Entamoeba polecki, 73
Epithelial cultures, 112
Erythrophagocytosis, 96
Evasion, of host defenses, 108
Excystation, 58,71
Exocytosis, 27-38,47

Filopodia, 8,10,42,44,49

Glucose, 61,69
Glycogen, 63,71
Glycolysis, 62
Glycoproteins, 66
Golgi system, 17
Growth and differentiation, 68

Immune reaction,
  cellular, 91
  humoral, 88
Immune serum, 89
Immunology, 85-93
Immunity, protective, 93
Immunoglobulins, 88
Immunosupression, 92
Indirect hemagglutination, 88
Inflammation, 111
Inorganic pyrophosphatase, 62
Invasive phase, 105
Iron, 105
Isoenzymes, 77,81,82,83

Karyosome, 50

Leukocytes, 103,111,112
Lipids, 65
Lobopodia, 8,42
Lymphocyte, mitogenic factors, 91
Lymphocytes, 91
Lysosomes, 12,13,17

Macrophages, 113,117
Macrophage, inhibiting factor, 91
Macropinocytosis, 8,12,25,38, 42
Membrane,
  antigens, 87
  composition, 65-67

Membrane - cont.
 freeze-fracture, 12,17,19,35, 44
 lipids, 65
 lysosomal, 13
 plasma, 12,13,17,32,35-42, 58
 vacuolar, 12,17
Metabolism, 61-64
Microexudate, 32,40,41
Microfilaments, 17,25,26
Micropinocytosis, 8,11,12,38,42
Microtubules, 11,25,26,55
Mitochondria, 11,61
Mitosis, 53
Monoclonal antibodies, 67,120
Motility, 107
Multiplication, 56,105
Myosin, 26

Nucleus, 26,50,58
Nuclear bodies, 50,51
Nuclear division, 53
Nuclear membrane, 50,51

Oxygen, 61,68,69

Pathogenic strains, 70,82,96, 117,119
Pathogenicity, 80,96
Penetration, 105
Phagocytosis, 17,27,42,61,107
Phospholipase, 66, 112
Phospholipoglycan, 65
Pinocytosis, 11,17,61
Polypeptides, 66
Proteins, 65,66,83
Pseudopodia, 10,11,38,42
Pyrophosphate, inorganic, 62, 63

Red blood cells, 11
Resistance to reinfection, 93

Ribosomal-like particles, 29
Rosettes, cytoplasmic, 27
RNA, 20,51

Serology, 89,92
Shedding, 32,40,90,108
Sialic acid, 35
Strain heterogeneity, 76-78, 102
Species of *Entamoeba*, 73,119
Surface-active lysosome, 47-49,112
Surface coat, 12,32-35,40,41, 44
Surface properties, 35,42,96, 97
Surface specializations, 42

Toxins, 19,109
Trophozoites, 5
Tubular system, 17

Uroid, 8,10,32,38,42,47

Vacuolar system, 11,12,13,17
Virulence, factors of, 95-117
Viruses,
 reoviruses, 26
 rhabdovirus-like, 29
 filamentous, 26,31
 polyhedral, 31
 virulence and, 31,98

Wall, cyst, 58,71

DATE DUE